Live FIT
From the Inside Out

The 6 SHIFTS to Living Your Strongest,
Healthiest, and Happiest Life

NICOLE ZAPOLI

Design and cover art by Mykhailo.

NIV: Scripture quotations taken from The Holy Bible, New International Version®, NIV®. Copyright © 1973, 1978, 1984, 2011 by Biblica, Inc. Used with permission of Zondervan.

Paperback ISBN: 978-1-967587-15-5
eBook ISBN: 978-1-967587-14-8

DEDICATION

For the family I was born into, the family I created, and the family I have met along my way—thank you for everything. I love you all.

For my clients. You all inspire me daily, more than you will ever know. Thank you for trusting me and allowing me to be part of your life.

For my first beautiful angel baby who made me a girl mommy, Rylee Grace—you are the most amazing, vibrant, fun, hardworking, intelligent young lady I know! Never change.

For my second beautiful angel baby who made me a boy mommy, Declan Makoa—your energy and laughter light up my life! Stay you.

For my best friend and soulmate, Jon—my favorite place is in your arms. Thank you for loving me in a way I didn't know I needed.

For every person, coach, client, and friend near and far who I have had the gift of knowing and having as part of my life's journey. I am so thankful for each of you in my life, whether it was for a season or you have been there my entire life. I would not be who I am today or where I am today without you.

CONTENTS

Be strong and courageous.
–Joshua 1:9 (NIV)

INTRODUCTION

I was 5 years old when my dad taught me how to do my first push-up. We were in the living room—him doing headstands, sit-ups, and push-ups—and me doing my best to copy every move. He coached me through each pushup, making sure I had the right form and technique, even at five. He wanted me to do it right...for that street cred, of course! What stuck with me wasn't just the physical strength I gained as a result—it was the pride I felt when I did it right, the joy of movement, and the quiet lesson he taught me about showing up for myself. That was my first taste of what it means to live fit.

HI, I'M NICOLE ZAPOLI!

I've worn many hats over the years, from competitive gymnast and professional cheerleader, professional dancer, and professional natural bodybuilder to CrossFit athlete, coach, and gym owner. With over 25 years of coaching experience in fitness and wellness, I've worked with people of all backgrounds to help them build strong, sustainable habits. My approach draws from a wide range of disciplines, including gymnastics, yoga, tactical and adaptive training, and physical therapy. Fitness and wellness aren't just what I do—they're who I am.

Today, I work with clients of all backgrounds and fitness levels to help them create long lives full of vitality and resilience. Through personalized fitness and nutrition coaching, I guide them in developing healthy routines that fit seamlessly into their lives. With that being said, this is NOT just another book about an exercise routine or diet. This book is all about practicing the consistent, sustainable lifestyle SHIFTS that produce lifelong results.

Fitness isn't about going to extremes or killing yourself trying to attain unreachable goals. At the same time, there is no quick fix or easy button for reaching those goals. Fitness is a lifestyle anyone can create, but to achieve it, you must take action and responsibility for your own health, life, and ultimately, your future. There are three things I believe are true for everyone, no matter where they're starting from.

First, anyone can improve their current level of fitness and wellness. There's this misconception that fitness has to look a certain way, or that it's something only an elite athlete can achieve. This simply is not true. Fitness is not some exclusive club. I wrote this book to emphasize that no matter where you're starting from and regardless of your background or age, it is possible for you to make changes that will transform your overall health, fitness, well-being, and quality of life for the long term. And this is true even if you have been actively fit for years—all of us have room to improve and to grow.

You also don't need a background in fitness, a fast metabolism, or a ton of free time. You just need to be willing to take action by creating your own simple, consistent daily lifestyle habits. Those clear, consistent investments in yourself on the daily add up and eventually are what lead to massive lifelong results. With a fundamental, step-by-step approach, you'll find that building a healthy, fulfilling life is completely within your reach.

Second, prioritizing your health is important. So often, I hear people say, "I wish I could do that, but…" and fill in the blank with any number of reasons. In fact, just a few months ago I had a booth at a fitness event for my fitness coaching business, NZ Fitness, and I heard something that almost broke my heart. As two women walked by my booth, one said to the other, "I wish I could work out, but I can't. I have kids."

I get it—life is busy, we have families, jobs, and responsibilities. But if we always put our health second, we will miss the chance to live life fully. Each individual has the power and ability to choose to change this. Putting your physical and mental health first will also help you to be an amazing example for your kids who will see you living out your own health and fitness journey day by day.

This book is here to help you eliminate those "buts" and turn them into "ands." Even as you shift in and out of different seasons in your life. Yes, you have a busy life—*and* you can still create a daily fitness and wellness routine that fits. Yes, you have kids—*and* you can be an amazing role model by showing them what's possible when you prioritize your health. I want to shift that mindset from "I *can't* because…" to "I *will* because…" In that way, you'll be creating a legacy of wellness that the people you love most can follow.

Third, you have the power to become stronger, healthier, and happier than you know! My ultimate goal for you isn't just for you to get fitter. I want you to start feeling strong and empowered in your own life. True fitness builds inner confidence and mental strength. When you discover what your body can do, from lifting a weight you never thought possible to running a mile without stopping, you begin to generate a respect for yourself that is powerfully life changing.

Let me be clear. Fitness and wellness are NOT about reaching a magic number on a scale or shrinking yourself down to a smaller dress size. They are about showing up and showing yourself what you're capable of. Every time you take a small step forward, you're building confidence, creating energy, and reinforcing the belief that you are strong and capable.

These truths are the reason I wrote this book—so that you can know what is possible for you and begin to work toward a stronger, healthier, happier life—no matter where you are in life right now.

THE SUPPORT YOU DIDN'T KNOW YOU NEEDED

This book is your stepping stone to beginning or reestablishing a lifelong fitness and wellness journey from where you are right now without feeling overwhelmed, getting burned out, or falling victim to the latest trendy fad diet. Inside, you'll learn the core SHIFTS you need to make in order to achieve better, more effective, sustainable outcomes like:

- Increased strength
- Improved energy and stamina
- More lean muscle mass
- Stronger mindset and mental resilience
- Less body fat

Overall, with this book, you'll have the blueprint to an improved quality of life through lifelong wellness. My goal for you is unwavering, long-term results that LAST. Now, let's go through a breakdown of how this book will help you achieve that.

This book is divided into three parts. First, I'll share the real story behind my own fitness and wellness journey—the highs, the lows, and the lessons that are not often shared or talked about. Then, I'll walk you through my SHIFTS Framework: six essential elements—sleep, hydration, intake, fitness, thoughts, and sunshine—that I've refined over 25+ years of coaching to help you get stronger mentally, emotionally, and physically. Finally, I'll show you how to put it all into action with goal-setting tools, movement tips, and practical resources, including some of my favorite NZ Fitness Meals and recipes, which you can find on this book's website, so you can build a lifestyle that fits you for the long haul.

Doesn't that sound like an adventure worth taking?

And, of course, if you want more personalized, guided support when it comes to mastering your fitness, wellness—and being accountable for your goals—I offer individually designed programs with one-on-one coaching available, both online and in person. Fill out the contact form on my website and I'll get back to you directly to book a call: https://nicolezapoli.com/contact/.

PART 1

Beyond Passion: Creating a Sustainable, Lifelong Journey in Fitness and Wellness

Chapter 1
Movement is Medicine

Movement has always been my anchor and my go-to when life feels overwhelming. It wasn't just about staying active. Movement was my therapy, my release, and my reset button. I never felt this more clearly than during my first pregnancy at age 22. I was in peak condition and fully expected to stay fit and active the whole way through. But by the end of my second trimester, things took a turn I didn't see coming.

My former husband and I were standing in line at Blockbuster getting ready for a fun movie night when I started having super close, consistent contractions. I went straight to my doctor to make sure my baby and I were safe. When my contractions didn't stop, my doctor put me on bed rest around the six-month mark. Suddenly, it felt as though my whole world shrank.

I've been active my whole life. Movement wasn't just something I did. It was how I lived.

When that happened in my pregnancy, all I was allowed to do was lie in bed or on the couch. Don't get me wrong—I would do anything to keep my baby safe and healthy. I followed my doctor's recommendations to a T, but staying still was incredibly hard. After a lifetime of daily movement, being confined to a couch felt like losing a part of myself. I did what I could—focused on my nutrition and did a ton of reading and journaling—but I missed feeling connected with my body. Thankfully, my doctor, a fit mom of five who understood my desire to move, eventually gave me the green light to ease back in with yoga, swimming, and walking a week or two before my due date.

My daughter was born safe and healthy, but the experience left a mark on me. I didn't realize just how deeply it affected me until 17 years later when I was pregnant with my son.

Once again, I started having constant, regular contractions at around the same time as in my first pregnancy. And once again, I found myself heading straight to my doctor to make sure everything was okay. I met with several medical professionals who immediately started throwing around words like "advanced maternal age" and "high risk." I knew that my age was a factor, but I also knew I was going into this pregnancy the fittest I'd ever been. Plus, this time around I was older, wiser, and had 17 years of experience training, coaching, and learning to listen to my body even more.

Instead of feeling powerless, this time I trusted my body, my mind, and the years of hard work I had put into understanding myself.

I checked in with my doctors, of course, and they did all the tests to make sure I wasn't in preterm labor. But I listened to my intuition, too, and my intuition told me that my baby and I were doing amazing. I kept moving in ways that felt good for my mental health and my changing body's needs, and I knew we would be okay.

Every day, I tuned into what my body needed. I always felt so much better after I got in some movement, so I maintained my training schedule consistently, as I had prepregnancy. I modified movement as needed. If a specific movement didn't feel right, I'd scale back or make adjustments. I became more attuned to my body than ever before, noticing subtle changes and learning to trust my inner compass. I kept moving all the way up to the day I went into labor––over two weeks past my original due date! I cannot tell you how amazing it was to not be lying in bed waiting for life to happen to me the whole time.

The difference between my first and second pregnancies was pretty dang profound. I am so grateful to have had the most miraculous experience of birthing two beautiful, healthy babies at the end of my pregnancies. That really is the most important thing. But while my first pregnancy felt like a period of confinement and restriction where I was forced into stillness, my second pregnancy was the complete opposite. I felt empowered, connected to my body, and oh so capable.

Movement was the medicine that helped me feel grounded and reminded me that pregnancy didn't have to mean forfeiting my strength.

Movement was an opportunity to honor and amplify that strength.

After that story, you might be wondering: Is movement medicine for you? If your answer is "yes", then you're going to love this book and the SHIFTS Framework!

If you haven't yet experienced movement as medicine, that is completely okay. I'll show you how to get started in this book. Or, if you want more movement as medicine, I have you covered. I am so super pumped for you to discover the SHIFTS that will move you towards your fitness and wellness goals!

WHAT DO I MEAN BY FITNESS AND WELLNESS?

Before we get any further into this book, I want to define what I mean when I use the words fitness and wellness. Many people hear these words and immediately think about losing weight or dropping dress sizes.

Are those things bad?

Heck no!

But, to me, fitness and wellness are not just about reaching a number on a scale or achieving a certain look. Fitness and wellness are about living with strength, confidence, and freedom in your own body, like I did in my second pregnancy. When you're fit and well, you can face every day feeling capable, resilient, and in control. Fitness and wellness are about cultivating lifestyle habits that support you, no matter your age or stage in life, so you can keep doing the things you love. True fitness and wellness means empowering yourself to live strong, healthy, and happy for the long haul.

Picture yourself hiking more mountains, playing with your kids, having newfound levels of energy, and having the vitality to conquer personal and professional goals.

Picture yourself the strongest, most flexible, and most energized you've ever been.

Picture yourself bursting with confidence knowing you did the work and are now reaping the rewards.

Picture yourself growing in mental toughness in all areas of your life!

That's the power of true fitness and wellness!

That's the power of making SHIFTS.

Sounds amazing, right? Who wouldn't want those things?

I've been a fitness and wellness coach for more than two decades and have worked with thousands of clients. I've competed in fitness competitions and professional sports at the highest levels since I was a kid.

This is my life.

You can believe me when I tell you that no matter who you are, what your background is, or where you're starting from, living fit, strong, healthy, and happy IS possible for you!

BUILD A STRONGER, HEALTHIER, AND HAPPIER YOU

Amazing things happen when you start showing up for yourself and begin taking consistent action to improve your overall fitness and wellness. Imagine waking up every morning feeling energized. Instead of dreading the day ahead, you'll know that no matter how busy or chaotic things get, you can handle them. Imagine having more playfulness, vigor, and stamina to keep up with your kids when they want to head to the park. Imagine changing your body composition by decreasing fat and increasing your lean muscle mass.

Fitness is about creating lasting change by showing up for yourself and doing what it takes to live a healthy, well-rounded lifestyle. When you start now and take essential, consistent steps, you will see a massive difference over time that results in a stronger, healthier, and happier you.

I call these simple, consistent steps "SHIFTS," and here's why…

Making progress is all about taking the step that's right in front of or even right next to you—and *continuing* on the path to lifelong fitness and wellness. Fitness and wellness aren't achieved by giant leaps. That is not sustainable, nor does it last. Seeing real change is all about making fundamental shifts consistently over time to achieve true longevity.

By now, you might be wondering what this looks like in real life and how making these shifts works for my clients— whether they're just starting their wellness and fitness journey or they want to take things to the next level. In the rest of this chapter, I'm going to share some stories of the results my clients experience using my SHIFTS Framework. I hope you'll see yourself in their stories and get excited about what is possible for you, too! An asterisk (*) indicates that a name has been changed to protect the individual's privacy.

CONSISTENT ACTION EQUALS ACTUAL RESULTS

Sophie*, age 40: From Injuries to 5% Less Body Fat

Sophie had been an athlete, dancer, and gymnast for most of her life. After years of pulling long office hours five days a week and having two kids, she felt like she had nothing left at the end of the day for herself. No energy, no motivation, and no time. On top of that, every time she tried to get active again, she kept aggravating an old lower-back injury. She felt like she was always in a "one step forward, two steps back" loop, and she was frustrated and discouraged.

Then a friend referred Sophie to me. She started incorporating my SHIFTS Framework into her daily life right away. Together, we came up with a fitness and wellness plan that didn't aggravate her old injury. She added more protein to her diet, which cut down on cravings and hunger. Sophie also got really serious about hydration, sleep, sunshine, and her mindset. After just a few months, here's what Sophie had to say:

"It has been about four months now, and I am down a noticeable amount of weight. I have added muscle, and I feel much stronger in my body. My lower back continues to accept the workouts for the most part with the strict attention to form that Nicole helps me with. I feel less like I need to hide parts of my body that have always bothered me. I think the best part of the whole endeavor is knowing that I CAN live an active lifestyle without ending up on the injured list all the time."

As of October 2024, Sophie had gained 1.5 pounds of lean mass, lost almost seven pounds, and reduced her body fat by 5%. By March 2025, she had continued to decrease her body fat percentage and lost nearly another seven pounds. These days, we have set a new goal to focus more on consistent daily protein and carb intake. She'll also be lifting heavier with more consistency so she can continue to build more lean mass while maintaining the already amazing progress she has achieved. I'm so proud of what Sophie has accomplished, and she is too!

Hadley Kelly, age 19: Achieving Big Goals

I first met Hadley at a bodybuilding show when she was just 17 years old. I was so impressed by her dedication to bodybuilding at such a young age, I couldn't resist getting a photo with her and spending a little time chatting with her about her fitness journey.

Hadley has big goals, but she also has a busy life as a college student and athlete. She was concerned about staying fit in a way that was sustainable year round, not just during competition season. She lived in fear of seeing the scale go up during the rest of the year, which broke my heart because I knew it did not have to be that way.

Together, Hadley and I created a plan focused on building lean muscle mass, not reaching a number on the scale. With the help of all six elements of my SHIFTS Framework, she quickly met her next goal. During this time, she also received a scholarship to play soccer at University of Texas Permian Basin. Today, Hadley is stronger than she's ever been and, at the time of this book, is preparing to compete in her next powerlifting and bodybuilding shows.

"I've realized that consistency is the most important tool. Prioritizing your nutrition and training will help you live longer and healthier. The happiness I have gained from my increased strength is immeasurable. I now look at fitness as a way to not only help yourself, but everyone in your life."

My favorite part of Hadley's story is how big her heart is! Not only does she take the SHIFTS Framework and run with it in her own life, she shares it with others so they can experience the benefits of a healthier lifestyle, too.

Larry, age 60: Out of a Slump and into Momentum

When I first met Larry, he was in a real fitness slump. He wasn't working out consistently, and when he did exercise, he did the same old workouts over and over again. Larry wasn't being challenged—in fact, he seemed to be a bit bored and was ready to shake things up.

Larry created a consistent fitness schedule along with hiring me as his trainer so he was more inclined to stay on track while moving in the direction he wanted to go—by incorporating variety in his training sessions to keep him building and progressing.

"I can now say that fitness is a regular part of my weekly life, and most of my days. Even on business trips, I now look forward to the gym at 6 am rather than the bar at 8 pm. I have a more toned body and my balance and strength have seriously improved over when I started."

Larry has been implementing the SHIFTS Framework for several years now, and the results are clear. Not only is he fitter, but his balance and strength have greatly improved. And perhaps, most important of all, he can now say that fitness is a regular part of his life.

Aaron*, age 40: Improved Health and Bloodwork in Four Months!

Aaron hadn't prioritized his health and fitness since having kids around eight years before we met. His family history of diabetes, cancer, arthritis, and heart disease seemed to hang over his head. He knew if he let his weight get out of control, that would be his future, too. He started by increasing his activity level by choosing to begin his day with an hour of activity and in just a few months, the results were remarkable. He also cut out a lot of the sweets, snacks, and carbs from his diet, substituting his old standby choices with new recipes that added variety to his meals.

"I am seeing physical results, such as a smaller waist, clothes fitting better, and increased definition. I also just feel less achy and 'old,' which allows me to enjoy time with my friends and family more."

Not only had Aaron transformed physically—as of October 2024, he had lost 11 pounds and 3% of his body fat—but also he feels more alert and ready to start his day. Plus, he can perform many exercises that he couldn't do when he started working with me, and he has more energy to be a better father, husband, and employee. Best of all, he's transforming his health right before his eyes. Within three months of starting to use the SHIFTS Framework, his blood work had improved over the year before. His cholesterol was down, and his A1C and all other markers were normal.

After the body composition measurements we did in October, our goal was to increase lean mass and not focus so much on body weight in pounds. He shifted his focus to fueling his body properly each day to hit his protein goals. He also challenged himself during his training sessions by lifting heavier weights on a more regular basis. By March 2025, he had gained two more pounds of lean muscle mass, lost three more pounds of body weight, and decreased his total body fat by 3%.

These clients have benefited greatly from using the SHIFTS Framework—wherever they were in their journeys—to make fitness and wellness parts of their daily lives. Imagine what it could do for you!

NOW, IT'S YOUR TURN!

Following SHIFTS gives you the path to build lifelong habits that will allow you to move in ways that actually support your life, while you learn how to maintain a solid balance and become empowered to make more precise health choices.

It's time to think about what could be possible for you if you went on a similar journey to what all of these amazing humans experienced!

By the time you finish reading this book, you will have every tool you need to take more action toward achieving longevity in a way that transforms your body, mind, and soul.

And, you'll be able to handle whatever comes your way—because that's what true health is!

It's more than just physical.

It's wellness from the inside out.

KEY TAKEAWAYS FROM CHAPTER 1

1. **Fitness and wellness are about living well for life.** It's not about the scale—it's about strength, energy, and supporting your whole self inside and out.
2. **Movement is medicine.** It grounds you, lifts your spirit, and helps you grow through the hard stuff. Whether you're rebuilding or thriving, movement brings you back to yourself.
3. **Consistency creates results.** You don't need perfect—just consistent, intentional action. Start small. Keep showing up. That's how change happens.
4. **The SHIFTS Framework works!** Clients of all ages and stages have found success using SHIFTS, and you can too.

Chapter 2

From Leotards to Lifelong Fitness

When I was 8 years old, I stood in front of my class on Career Day with one of my competition leotards and warm-up suit on and boldly declared, "I'm going to be a coach and own my own gym." I was just a kid, and I didn't know how my dream would take shape, but I had 100% confidence that fitness and wellness would direct my path. I knew I was meant to lead people towards stronger, healthier, happier lives.

Like I said in Chapter 1, my love of fitness and wellness started young. My mom signed me up for dance at age 2 and artistic gymnastics at age 4. I entered competition at age 6, eventually transitioned to rhythmic, and by the time I was 14, I was training at the Olympic Training Center in Colorado. It wasn't all sunshine and rainbows though. For the first time, I was living and training eight-plus hours a day with other athletes—many who struggled with eating disorders. This was a different side of the sport I loved, and it opened my eyes to a need I hoped I could help meet someday.

Rhythmic gymnastics favors a body type with long lines. I'm not built like that, but it didn't bother me. Thankfully, even as a teen, I was confident in myself and with my body, and I've never felt the need to have to go to extreme measures to achieve a certain look. Not everyone has that confidence though, especially as a teen. My heart broke for my friends who'd developed severe eating disorders. But at the Olympic Training Center, staff members were doing something to help by requiring all athletes to attend nutrition classes, and I was all in.

My love for proper nutrition started in my childhood. My dad grew up on a farm in Michigan, and he was an amazing gardener and chef! When I was a kid, we had a mini farm in our backyard, and he built me my own planter. I learned how to plant seeds and nurture fruits and vegetables from the ground to the table. It was such a fun and empowering experience to know that I had grown my own food and could eat it!

When I saw the emphasis the Olympic Training Center's coaches and staff put on nutrition, it clicked! Fitness plus nutrition coaching…I could see myself doing that not just for a moment, but for the rest of my life! I could teach people the skills and practices that would help them reach their full potential not just physically, but mentally too—and I could support them as they worked to achieve lifelong fitness and wellness.

That's when I knew coaching wasn't just a dream—it was my path.

The declaration I made at age 8 and the decision I made at age 14, shaped everything about who I would become. Today, I am a professional fitness and wellness coach and certified personal trainer. I have been a fitness business owner and have owned multiple gyms for the past 25 years. I have worked with everyone from 19-year-old collegiate athletes and former professional athletes to busy professionals, active parents, and postpartum moms. I've also worked with kids of all ages all the way to adults 90+ years old, including military, first responders, and law enforcement officers. I've helped clients prep for fitness shows and competitions, reduce body fat and increase lean muscle mass, and improve their bloodwork and overall health. We've worked together to increase stamina and flexibility.

I am also a lifelong athlete. I work and train hard to stay in top condition, and I take a ton of pride in practicing what I preach. I'm involved in the competitive fitness world and have competed at a high level, setting records and winning awards in powerlifting, Olympic weightlifting, CrossFit, calisthenics, and professional natural bodybuilding.

Coaching isn't just my job. It's the heartbeat of my life, and I'm so glad you're here today reading this book because I'd love for our time together in these pages to be part of your fitness and wellness journey!

WHO IS THIS BOOK FOR?

This book is for people who are ready to take ownership of their health and overall quality of life. It's for people who want to achieve longevity and improve their quality of life through fitness and wellness in a holistic way. This is for anyone—whether you're an athlete, busy parent, or professional—who feels that their health goals have been out of reach. Those who are now ready to make lasting and meaningful changes.

You could be an athlete with big goals—a competition or season you want to excel in—and you're after targeted results that come from dialing in on a fitness and wellness regimen that can benefit you for a lifetime.

Maybe you've been active and fit your whole life, but you know there's more you want to achieve. You're ready to take things to the next level, but you want to do that in an informed and empowered way so the transformation you experience is lifelong.

Perhaps you've experienced a setback or break in your fitness regimen and you're ready to get back on track with a system that's meant for long-term, sustainable results.

Maybe you've tried making improvements on your fitness and wellness before, but felt overwhelmed by the sheer volume of information out there. Where do you start? How do you make sure you're progressing safely and consistently?

Perhaps you've used excuses like "I'm too busy" or "I have kids, so I don't have time" to put your health on the back burner. You might feel frustrated or even a bit ashamed when you see others leading the lifestyle you wish for. But you're also hopeful. You're ready to stop letting circumstances dictate your life and start making your well-being a priority.

If any of those statements above resonate with you, this book holds the key to making the consistent, sustainable shifts that will help you build a stronger, healthier, happier you.

And it will work for you...

Even if you live a crazy busy lifestyle and have had trouble sticking to something long term.

Even if you feel like you've been out of shape for too long.

Even if you're a beginner to the fitness world.

This book *isn't* for everyone though.

If you're reading this book right now hoping for a quick fix, extreme weight loss program, or are only interested in achieving a certain aesthetic instead of focusing on overall wellness or athletic performance, this book probably isn't what you're looking for.

If you only want cardio-based workouts or a calorie restriction plan for weight loss, that's not what my framework will do for you.

BUT if you're a person who's looking for a holistic approach to fitness and wellness that impacts body, mind, and soul, you're in the right place. If you're ready to say, "Yes, I can prioritize myself. I can be a parent *and* take care of my health," I've got the exact framework you need to make changes step by step and stick to those changes.

AND if you're looking to create the life you want without sacrificing your own well-being, keep reading because you're going to love the simple, sustainable approach I teach.

WHAT DOES THIS MEAN FOR YOU?

This book is about YOU, and I want you to know how serious I am about helping people create a lifelong, high-quality fitness and wellness lifestyle. You don't have to be a super fitness fanatic like I am to reap the benefits of a stronger, healthier, happier life. Fitness and wellness will help you gain the independence to move through life with energy and freedom, whether that means trying a new physical activity, being ready for your next show or competition, or simply living with minimal to no limitations as you age.

No matter what your experience with fitness and wellness has been in the past, your health and well-being are within your control. This approach is not just about strengthening your body. It's about building strength mentally, too, and finding empowerment in what your body can do. I do what I do so my clients can know and experience the joy of accomplishing something they didn't think was possible, whether it's their first pull-up, a personal record in a workout or lift, or the confidence and pride to show up for themselves every day.

Fitness teaches and develops discipline and consistency, and those habits create true transformation. It's not about quick fixes or crash diets. It's about making lasting changes, one step at a time, in a way that enables you to live the life you want filled with energy, resilience, and the ability to keep doing the things you love for years to come.

When you prioritize fitness and wellness, you're setting yourself up to live a high-quality life where you can stay active so you don't have to rely on others as much as you age.

It's about teaching and leading your kids by example and breaking free from the excuses that may be keeping you stuck. Taking care of yourself is one of the most empowering things you can do, and it ripples out into every part of your life.

This isn't just another fitness book. If you're looking for the latest workout of the week, that's not what you'll find here.

Will I share body weight training based on functional gymnastic movements anyone can do and fitness tips like the ones I share with my clients?

Heck yes!

But I'll also be teaching you about fitness and wellness foundations like hydration, sleep, sunshine, and mindset. Each of these core elements that I call SHIFTS plays a part in helping you live your strongest, healthiest, happiest life.

The bottom line is, what I'm offering you, in these pages, is a roadmap to transformation, inside and out, that's doable and sustainable for the long term. And we're going to do it together, one shift at a time.

SO...WHAT'S NEXT?

If this chapter resonates with you, it's time to make a decision. The most powerful thing you can do right now to move closer to your fitness and wellness goals is to commit to showing up for yourself by reading through this book and implementing the SHIFTS as you learn them.

It won't be an overnight transformation. Programs that promise quick change and near-instant results are not sustainable, and the results do not last.

That is not what I'm after for you.

In contrast to those false promises that offer you dramatic results in no time at all, my SHIFTS Framework is something you can take with you throughout the *rest of your life* and pass on to your children, share with your friends and family members, and feel good about when you lay your head down on your pillow at night.

I'll be breaking the entire SHIFTS Framework down step by step in Part 2 of this book, but here's a quick summary of what you can expect. As you read this book, I'll give you my roadmap to lifelong fitness and wellness in a way that is doable and customizable to *your* reality, not someone else's ideals. Inside, you'll find guidance that goes deeper than quick fixes, gimmicks, or crash diets. Plus, I'm including a bunch of tools and resources on the book's website to help you track your progress as you build strength, improve your health, and gain confidence.

My goal for you is that before you even finish reading, you will have redefined what fitness and wellness mean for you. You'll be empowered in your body, mind, and soul, and confident in your ability to reach your goals, setting an example for your children and the fellow fitness enthusiasts and athletes in your circle.

Throughout Part 1 of this book, you'll come across a few self-assessments. These assessments will help you get the most out of this book by prompting you to take a deeper look at where you are today and where you want to be as you move forward. As we wrap up this chapter, take a moment to fill out your very first self-assessment below.

SELF-ASSESSMENT: ARE YOU READY TO TRANSFORM?

Read each statement below and answer True or False:

I am dissatisfied with my current fitness level and know I can do better.

- True
- False

I feel the need to make a lifestyle shift to improve my overall quality of life.

- True
- False

I am ready to commit to consistent action toward my health and wellness goals.

- True
- False

I recognize that my current habits may not be serving my long-term well-being.

- True
- False

I understand that progress takes time, and I am willing to stay the course.

- True
- False

I am open to learning, adapting, and challenging myself in new ways.

- True
- False

I want to build strength—not just physically, but mentally and emotionally as well.

- True
- False

I know that the best investment I can make is in myself.

- True
- False

If you answered "True" to most or all of these, this book is for you! Now, take a moment to define your vision:

» Who are you becoming this year? (Write it down. Clarity creates momentum.)

» What actions will reinforce that identity? (Success is built on daily decisions. List the ones you plan to take.)

KEY TAKEAWAYS FROM CHAPTER 2

1. **Fitness + wellness = lifestyle.** I didn't just "get into" fitness—I grew up in it. From living room push-ups to dreaming of owning a gym at 8 years old, this has always been my path. This chapter will help you adopt the same mindset so your results last for life.

2. **Nourishment is a gift.** I learned early how food connects to wellness—gardening with my dad, cooking from scratch. When you treat food and fitness with intention, everything changes.

3. **Coaching is my calling.** I've coached thousands—from pros to new moms. No matter your age, schedule, or past—today is a great day to begin.

4. **This book is for you.** Whether you're a mom, an athlete, or starting over (again), you belong here. Fitness isn't just for the elite—it's a tool for living well on your terms.

5. **SHIFTS is your roadmap.** Sleep, Hydration, Intake, Fitness, Thoughts, and Sunshine—the six daily habits that create lasting change. You'll learn how to make them part of your life for good.

Chapter 3

Mindset Minefields

The toughest seasons in my life have brought about the most profound growth. I have learned that I see the greatest results on the other side of an experience when I choose to dig deep, push through, and do the work. And I'm not just talking about physical transformation. The body and the mind are deeply connected.

That's never been more obvious to me than when I started doing CrossFit—a method of training defined as "constantly varied functional movements performed at high intensity."[1] I was at a point in my life where I was managing and balancing multiple responsibilities and demands with running my business, raising my young daughter, and navigating being a newly single mom. Before I started CrossFit, I didn't know much about it. I just knew I needed something for *me*.

With CrossFit, you never know what you're going to get from workout to workout. You might see anything from handstand walks, to pull-ups, to push-ups, to sprints, to wall balls, to squats, to deadlifts, to cleans, and more. Every workout was a test of both my physical and mental strength because I had never been pushed quite like that before. I wasn't new to tough challenges, but CrossFit took things to a whole new level. I decided to embrace the discomfort and keep moving forward, despite how tough it was.

It wasn't just about showing up for the workout.

It was about showing up for myself.

Was it hard? Heck yes.

Some days I felt strong, and others I had to modify movements to meet myself where I was. Learning to trust my body's signals became as important as completing the workout.

Although I noticed an almost immediate physical change in my body, what surprised me even more was the mental strength I developed. CrossFit became more than just exercise—it was a way for me to continue to level up and build more discipline and resilience. It helped me reframe how I approach challenges in life. I learned to adjust, stay consistent, and find strength in the process. Over time, I saw myself grow even more in confidence, too.

The physical and mental benefits and rewards I've received from being involved in CrossFit far outweigh any of my competitive achievements. CrossFit taught me to focus on what I have the power to control—my mindset—and to trust my body while finding joy in the process.

If you're reading this book right now, you know you need to start making changes that will lead to longevity through fitness and wellness. When you do, it's not only your physical condition that will give you pushback. It's your mindset. And, as a result of dedicated training, it's not just your physical condition that will benefit. Your mindset will benefit, too.

The amazing thing is, moving your body is what your mind needs, and science proves it! A recent study of university students linked outdoor activity with improved mood, focus, and comprehension. It found that when the students replaced ten minutes of sitting with ten minutes of outdoor physical activity, it boosted their moods and mental clarity significantly![2] This indicates that getting in some movement prior to reading, studying, or listening to a lecture increases a person's ability to focus, comprehend, and retain new information.

In this chapter, I break down some of the things that might be running through your mind right now—some of the hurdles you may face as you prepare to get started. Then, after each hurdle, you'll find a self-assessment to complete. These assessments will help you pinpoint which hurdles you may be facing. You'll also learn how my SHIFTS Framework will help you overcome these hurdles so you can live YOUR strongest, healthiest, happiest life possible.

HURDLE #1: "I CAN'T START UNTIL/BECAUSE..."

When people first start their fitness and wellness journeys, they often walk into it carrying the weight of their own limiting beliefs—and that can be super heavy! Limiting beliefs will impact your progress, so you must leave those limiting beliefs behind so they don't sideline your goals and dreams of longevity and lifelong fitness and wellness. Here are some of the most common limiting beliefs I hear as a coach and trainer.

"I can't start until I'm in better shape."
Many people assume they need to look a certain way or be able to do ten push-ups or run a mile without stopping before they can get started. Sometimes they sign up for an inexpensive gym membership, thinking they'll embrace fitness and wellness on their own, but without help or guidance and accountability, they get discouraged and give up when they don't see results. Sound familiar?

The Truth: Just start. Everyone—every athlete you admire, every coach you trust—had a day one. You can choose to believe whatever limiting beliefs you face and stay stuck for another month, six months, two years, or the rest of your life. *Or* you can take small, consistent steps forward. These steps don't have to be perfect or even dramatic. Maybe it's walking into a CrossFit gym three days a week. Just being there and showing up can lead to incredible results over time.

Consistency, even in the simplest actions, is where the magic happens. Day by day, each tiny win adds up. If you're unsure how to begin, use this book as your guide. Walk chapter by chapter through my SHIFTS Framework. Start with what you can do now, and grow as you go. You won't transform overnight, but every time you take action, no matter how small, it solidifies your commitment, increases your belief, and contributes to your overall and lifelong transformation. Over time, this impacts who you are, who you will be tomorrow, and who you will be at the end of your life.

You don't have to overhaul your life overnight. If you need help, consider having me design a personalized training program with remote coaching for you specifically. There are always ways to add movement into your life, and you can start today.

But what if pain or fear from a past injury is holding you back?

You are not alone!

"I can't start because of an old injury."

Past injuries can make it hard to stay fit while keeping a positive mindset. Just remember, you're injured, not broken. Don't give in to the temptation to succumb to victim status. It's common to worry about reinjury and be reluctant to risk it. It's hard to trust your body again after an injury, especially one that plays over and over in your mind. This fear keeps people stuck.

The Truth: Coming back from an injury will be tough at first. You might feel like you'll never get back to where you were prior to your injury. Depending on the severity of your injury, fitness may never look quite the same for you, and that's okay. Don't let that stop you from working toward the best version of you, today.

You might not be able to change what happened, but you CAN reframe how you think about your injury. I love how James Clear talks about changing the story you tell about difficult things that happened previously in your life. "You can't change your past, but you can reframe it. Find the lesson in it. Find the opportunity in it. Pull the teachable moment out of it and share it with others. You can't choose your history, but you can choose the story you tell about it."[3]

Your body is more adaptable than you think. Start small by learning or relearning proper technique and form. Give your body time to adapt and trust the process. That trust between your mind and body doesn't come overnight, but as you practice consistently, you'll start to feel the connection grow stronger.

And don't mistake muscle soreness for injury. That's your body's way of telling you it's growing stronger. Make sure you're paying attention to your recovery. Stretch, move gently, and keep going. The results—living stronger and longer—are worth that kind of muscle soreness.

"I can't start because of a disability."
The Truth: Having a disability doesn't mean you can't live your strongest, healthiest, happiest life. It just might look different than you expected. Whether it's adaptive athletes, individuals with disabilities, including those with visible and invisible injuries like traumatic brain injuries or post-traumatic stress disorder, their stories show what's possible when you focus on what you can do rather than on what you can't. Watching these remarkable humans embrace movement and push beyond what others might believe possible, or label as limitations, has been nothing short of life changing for me.

One client I worked with had been told that his physical challenges would prevent him from living an active life. He refused to believe that, and instead we focused on movement that worked for his body. He started with small steps—

mobility exercises and strengthening the muscles he could control. Over time, I watched as he not only grew stronger, but began to see himself differently. It wasn't just about the physical progress. It was about the mental transformation. Movement gave him confidence, a sense of control, and the independence that he thought he had lost.

I've had the privilege of working with a client who had a stroke that affected one entire side of his body. I've also had the opportunity to work with athletes and clients who are amputees. We worked hard to create and modify movement that allowed them to improve their fitness safely and effectively, while maintaining and achieving proper form and technique. It's about showing up and believing in your own ability to keep leveling up and moving forward and know your worth.

These experiences have shaped how I approach fitness and wellness. Movement isn't just for the elite or for those without physical limitations. Fitness and wellness are for everyone. It's about staying consistent, finding what works for you, and embracing the process. Seeing people take ownership of their own health, adapt to challenges, and discover their inner strength reminds me that the possibilities are endless when you choose to see obstacles as opportunities rather than roadblocks.

SELF-ASSESSMENT: ARE LIMITING BELIEFS MY HURDLE?

Read each statement and answer True or False:

I often tell myself, "I can't" before I've even tried.

- True
- False

I avoid new challenges because I assume I won't be good at them.

- True
- False

When I face an obstacle, my first instinct is to step back rather than push forward.

- True
- False

I believe I need to be in better shape before starting a structured fitness program.

- True
- False

I worry that past injuries will prevent me from making progress.

- True
- False

I've put off working on my fitness or wellness goals for months (or years).

- True
- False

I compare myself to others and feel like I'll never measure up.

- True
- False

I sometimes feel like small steps aren't worth the effort unless they create instant results.

- True
- False

When things get uncomfortable, I tend to quit rather than adapt.

- True
- False

I struggle to trust my body's ability to adapt and get stronger.

- True
- False

If you answered "True" to several of these, you may be holding onto limiting beliefs that are keeping you stuck. Now, take a moment to flip the script.

What's one belief from above that you can rewrite into an empowering statement?
(Example: Instead of "I can't because of an old injury," try "I can modify my workouts and move in ways that support my body.")

What's one action you can take today to show yourself that you can?

Starting a fitness journey begins with mindset first. When you realize you can overcome discomfort and push through hard moments, you begin to see how mental strength carries over into every area of your life. You don't have to allow limiting beliefs to hold you back. Rely on the SHIFTS Framework in this book to provide the road map, start where you are, and trust yourself. The journey isn't just about physical fitness— it's about discovering the strength you already have within yourself to do hard things.

HURDLE #2: "I DON'T HAVE TIME."

"I don't have enough time" or "I don't have time because I have kids" are some of the most common reasons I hear people give for not keeping to a fitness and wellness regimen.

Busy life? Oh, I hear you. Busy feels like a baseline for so many of us. I'm living it, too, as a mom, a partner, coaching a full roster of clients both in person and online, and growing my business with roots in San Diego and connections far beyond. I am also training for multiple events. So yes, life is full. But I have come to see movement and wellness not as something I squeeze in, but as something I make space for and something that steadies me. It helps me show up better in all areas. It's not one more thing on the list. It is what helps me carry it all while staying true to who I am and honoring the best version of myself.

The Truth: People make time for the things that matter to them. You will find time for fitness when you choose to make it a priority. That's why the first step I take people through in my SHIFTS Framework is how to create space in their lives for fitness.

You have to schedule it, then honor and keep the commitment you make to yourself and your health, and I'll show you exactly how to do that in chapter 5. Prioritizing your health gives you more—and better quality—time. Not only will you be bettering your health long term and increasing your longevity, you'll be modeling the importance of fitness and wellness for your kids. For me, anytime I train, it helps me grow as a person, as a mom, as a trainer, and as a business owner/entrepreneur.

When you schedule your workouts, it becomes a part of your life and part of who you are—which will in turn help you rise up and overcome the inevitable stresses we all face. Now look at your situation using the self-assessment below to determine whether time is a hurdle for you.

SELF-ASSESSMENT: IS TIME MY HURDLE?

Read each statement and answer True or False:

My to-do list is never ending, and I often feel like I didn't accomplish enough.

- True
- False

My schedule is so packed that I struggle to find time for myself.

- True
- False

I believe a workout only "counts" if it exceeds a certain length of time.

- True
- False

I frequently put others' needs ahead of my own, leaving little time for my health.

- True
- False

I often tell myself, "I'll start when things slow down."

- True
- False

I feel guilty taking time for myself when there's so much to do.

- True
- False

I prioritize work and responsibilities over movement and self-care.

- True
- False

If you answered "True" to several of these, time may be your biggest hurdle.

Reframing Your Mindset

Choose one statement you answered "True" to and rewrite it into an empowering belief. (Example: Instead of "I'll start when things slow down," try "I can start with small, consistent actions even in busy seasons.")

What's one way you can create or protect time to prioritize your health this week?

Your fitness and wellness won't take care of themselves. The good news is, it's not as time consuming as you might think to prioritize these parts of life, and the benefits are endless! Don't buy the lies that you have to drive an hour to the gym or spend multiple hours in the gym at every session. You can get amazing results with as little as 30 minutes of activity three or more times per week. An effective fitness program, proper nutrition and lifestyle habits, and a strong mindset make a lasting impact on your health and quality of life. All you need is a commitment to taking consistent action on the SHIFTS you'll learn in this book.

HURDLE #3: "IT'S NOT THE PERFECT TIME YET."

Another hurdle people face when they're thinking about starting a lifelong fitness and wellness journey is the idea that everything has to be perfect before you start. Starting something new can be intimidating. It's easier to put things off until conditions are exactly "perfect," but if you do, you will most likely never start.

The Truth: There is no such thing as the "perfect" time to start anything, including a fitness and wellness plan. There is only now, and your future self is waiting for you to show up for her or him today! If you're stuck on the idea that you don't want to look silly or that you'll have to perform up to a certain level right away, let those ideas go, too. Everyone goes through this season of wanting perfection on some level, but you are capable of rising above it.

I once heard a story about this from one of my past coaches. He told me that training is like moving a huge pile of dirt. Some days you get a shovel, and some days you get a spoon. The important thing is to use what you have in that moment to move a little bit of the dirt each day. That will keep you moving in the right direction.

SELF-ASSESSMENT: IS PERFECTIONISM MY HURDLE?

Read each statement and answer True or False:

I avoid trying new things unless I'm confident I'll be good at them.

- True
- False

If I can't do something perfectly, I often won't do it at all.

- True
- False

When I fall short of my expectations, I feel frustrated or discouraged.

- True
- False

I set high standards for myself that sometimes feel impossible to meet.

- True
- False

I struggle to celebrate small wins because I focus on what still needs improvement.

- True
- False

If I miss a workout or eat something that's off my plan, I feel like I've failed.

- True
- False

I get stuck in planning mode, waiting for the "perfect" time to start.

- True
- False

Once I have an ideal outcome in mind, it's hard to adjust my expectations.

- True
- False

I often compare my progress to others and feel like I'm behind.

- True
- False

I don't like to embrace small, consistent steps when progress isn't immediate.

- True
- False

If you answered "True" to several of these, perfectionism may be holding you back.

REFRAMING YOUR MINDSET

Choose one statement you answered "True" to and rewrite it into an empowering belief. (Example: Instead of "If I can't do something perfectly, I often don't do it at all," try "Progress, not perfection, is the goal. Every step counts.")

What's one imperfect action you can take this week to move forward?

If perfectionism is in your way and keeping you stuck, my SHIFTS Framework is your call out and your breakthrough. It will help you overcome this hurdle by showing you how to commit to action, even when it's messy. And also how to keep showing up. Being perfectly fit isn't the goal, nor is it possible. There are always opportunities for growth when it comes to your fitness and wellness. Instead, focus on showing up for yourself, building your strength foundation, and continuing to make progress.

Don't forget that your mental health, strength, and resilience are powerful allies that help you to keep going, to conquer challenges, to breakthrough barriers, and to take charge of your fitness, health, and overall quality of life. Every step you take now—no matter how insignificant it might feel—builds a stronger, healthier, and happier future for yourself. The sooner you get going, the more you'll be able to invest in the mental and physical well-being, strength, and resilience of your future self. The longer you put off getting started because things aren't "perfect," the more you're stealing physical AND mental health, strength, and resilience from the future you.

But what if you have been putting in the time, yet it seems like your results have stalled? Let's look at the next hurdle.

HURDLE #4: "I'VE HIT A PLATEAU."

Sometimes past experience can hold you back from wanting to keep going or to attempt trying again. When you try something and don't get the result you want—or your results taper off—it's hard to want to keep trying. In the fitness world, this is called "hitting a plateau" or "plateauing."

Plateaus can be physical or mental, and the mental ones are especially tricky because you may not even be aware of the subconscious blocks holding you back. You may feel as though you have worked through a ton of the mindset stuff and have made a ton of progress. Yet for some reason, you are just not able to make it past a certain level no matter how hard you work or how much you try to push through.

Mental plateaus go deep into the neurological side of fitness and underscores how important our brain health is. Working with a neurologist can help with overcoming your plateaus or limitations. You may also consider investing in a life coach who is trained at helping you break through those subconscious blocks or limiting beliefs.

The Truth: Hitting a plateau is more often the result of falling into your comfort zone and not challenging yourself. When you know how to vary your workouts and embrace discomfort rather than staying in your comfort zone, it's pretty hard to plateau.

SELF-ASSESSMENT: IS THE COMFORT ZONE MY HURDLE?

Are you stuck in the comfort zone? Answer the questions below.

Do you consistently train each week? Y/N

Do you consistently train at or around a 6–8 in terms of exertion on a scale of 1–10, with 1 being a casual stroll and 10 being maximum exertion? Y/N

Do you periodically challenge yourself to go heavier than the week or month before? Y/N

Do you consistently embrace doing more challenging movement variations or mastering proper form and technique (rather than sloppily moving through superfast just to be done)? Y/N

Do you show up for training sessions to do bare minimum and make yourself feel better that you showed up, rather than putting in actual effort and some solid work? Y/N

Do you consistently track and log your daily training? Y/N

Do you reference back to your log to retest baselines and previous repeat workouts to measure your progress? Y/N

How often do you check your body composition?

If you think you've hit a plateau, it sounds like it's time for a shift! This book is just what you need to shake things up a bit and break out of the fitness or wellness plateau you've found yourself on. In chapter 7, I'll lead you through all six SHIFTS and show you how to create a personalized plan to get back on track. You'll learn how to:

- Track your workouts and results
- Get back on the consistency train if you fall off
- Recommit to taking simple, consistent action
- Reframe your mindset around setbacks and comfort zones

But even with a clear plan and fresh motivation, one of the biggest challenges many people face isn't actually the workout—it just might be the people around them.

HURDLE #5: "MY FRIENDS AND FAMILY AREN'T SUPPORTIVE. I'M AFRAID THEY'LL JUDGE ME."

Not everyone will understand your desire for lifelong fitness and wellness. For some people, your desire for a healthy life might make them feel guilty about their unhealthy habits. Not everyone will support you. Some will question your choices and act as though you're doing something wrong. Yes, it can be frustrating, but it also says more about them than it does you.

Just know this: You're not walking this path alone.

I got married at the age of 18 years old after the pastor of the local youth group I was part of told my youth-pastor boyfriend and I that it was God's will that we get married.

I had so many dreams for my life—dreams of college, competitive cheer, dance, and opening my own gym—and I had the talent. In competitive cheer alone, I was a three-time All-American and nominated my senior year of high school for the National Cheerleading Association staff, one of only three others selected out of thousands. They told me they had been scouting me for years. Marriage wasn't even on my radar.

But out of fear of letting someone down, especially God, I got married.

Within a year of getting married, the opportunity came up for me to try out to be an NFL cheerleader for the Houston Texans. I was so excited. The NFL—this was one of my dreams! Before I tried out, my then-husband asked our church's pastor for permission. He was concerned about how my being an NFL cheerleader would be perceived within the church community, especially with me being the youth pastor's wife. The pastor agreed I could try out, so I did.

I made the squad, which was a huge accomplishment! I was thrilled, but instead of being happy and excited for me, the same pastor who had granted his "permission" changed his tune. When I told him I'd made it, he referred to NFL cheerleaders as "glorified prostitutes" and insisted I could only be on the team for one year. He treated my achievement as if my success was something shameful to be tolerated rather than celebrated. He even admitted that he'd only agreed because he never thought I would make it.

The hardest part, though, was how the women in our church—women I considered my closest friends—turned on me. They sat me down intervention-style and told me that by wanting to be an NFL cheerleader and trying out, I had a deep-seated sin issue and needed to repent. These were women I hoped would be my biggest support team, and instead they became my harshest critics, leaving me isolated and heartbroken.

Sometimes in life, the people you hope will be your biggest supporters and sources of unconditional love and strength—the ones you should be able to trust more than anyone—end up proving to be the exact opposite. That kind of betrayal is gut-wrenching and can leave you stunned, heartbroken, and questioning everything.

I hope you've never experienced anything like this or felt the way these comments and experiences made me feel. But if you have, just know you are NOT alone, and you can get through these types of circumstances.

The Truth: Not everyone will understand you and your way of life. Not everyone will support your dreams, even those you expect to be in your corner. Other people's doubts don't have to dictate your future. If anything, those doubts have the power to ignite an even fiercer fire to fuel you to pursue your dreams and goals.

It's so tough when the people in your life aren't supportive. The closer our relationship to those people, the harder it is to separate ourselves from allowing their words and opinions to affect us. James Clear explains why in his book *Atomic Habits: An Easy & Proven Way to Build Good Habits & Break Bad Ones* when he writes:

The more deeply a thought or action is tied to your identity, the more difficult it is to change it. It can feel comfortable to believe what your culture believes (group identity) or to do what upholds your self-image (personal identity), even if it's wrong. The biggest barrier to change at any level—individual, team, society—is identity conflict. Good habits can make rational sense, but if they conflict with your identity, you will fail to put them into action.[3]

The truth is, you don't have control over what other people say, think, or do. The most important thing is for you to do what makes you proud of yourself. Your fitness and wellness is important and deserves to be a priority in your life, so if you don't have support in your existing circle, find it in other settings like online training groups and fitness centers. If it gets to the point where the naysayers in your life are affecting your ability to stay consistent, don't hesitate to set some boundaries. As John Welbourn, founder and CEO of Power Athlete, says, "If you are the sum of the small circle of people you hang out with, you better have an interesting circle. If the circle sucks, change it quick."[4]

In the end, you must have the audacity, courage, and strength to bet on yourself wholeheartedly. You can create your own sense of peace and find contentment on your own terms. When you're down, you can get back up and keep charging forward.

As you read through the hurdles I described in this chapter, I hope you noticed that my solutions to them all are centered around functional fitness with a strong focus on mobility and bodyweight exercises, plus a deep mind-body connection. You won't learn a diet-of-the-month or the latest fitness workout fad here. Those things won't help you achieve lifelong fitness and wellness and a better quality of life in a way that is sustainable and doable for a lifetime.

My goal is that this book becomes your ultimate tool to creating a holistic and balanced fitness and wellness routine—for life. One where consistency over time, along with proper nutrition and mental resilience, play critical roles in achieving lifelong health and independence. In the next chapter, I'm going to reveal the one thing that will impact your results more than anything else—showing up for yourself. It really is the first, most important step to everything!

KEY TAKEAWAYS FOR CHAPTER 3

1. **Start small.** You don't need to know everything to begin. Just take one simple step. Progress comes from action, not perfection.
2. **Use what you've got.** A ten-minute walk or deep breaths matter. It's not about time—it's about intention.
3. **Find support.** You're not meant to do this alone. Community and accountability make the journey lighter and more fun.
4. **Keep going.** Consistency isn't perfection. Just keep showing up—even if you've missed a few days. That's how resilience is built.
5. **You belong here.** Fitness is for everyone. Don't let a bad experience or toxic culture keep you from finding a

welcoming space and supportive community. You don't
have to look a certain way to show up.

6. **It's okay to start again.** If you've stopped before, you're
not alone. This journey isn't about punishment for any
habits you fell out of—it's about building a real-life,
sustainable lifestyle that lasts.

---

[1] https://www.crossfit.com/what-is-crossfit

[2] Genevive R.Meredith, Gen, et al. "As Little as 10 Minutes in a Natural Setting Helps College Students Feel Happier and Lessens the Effects of Both Physical and Mental Stress," *Frontiers in Psychology*, Jan. 2020.

[3] James Clear, *Atomic Habits: An Easy & Proven Way to Build Good Habits & Break Bad Ones*, (Avery, 2018).

[4] John Welbourn, "If you are the sum of the small circle of people you hang out with…" *Power Athlete HQ*, accessed July 29, 2025. https://powerathletehq.com

Chapter 4

The Power of Self-Worth

Do not speak bad of yourself. For the warrior
within hears your words and is lessened by them.

-ancient Japanese proverb

I admit it—I used to have a relentless inner analyst and critic. Growing up, I was a people pleaser. I learned to make people happy, even if it meant silencing parts of myself. I came from a big, close-knit Italian family on my dad's side. I have loved and always looked forward to our family get-togethers ever since I was a little girl. They were super fun, and I still love spending time with family. So, I found it super strange when I experienced post get-together anxiety.

Everyone was involved in each other's lives, and looking back, I can see I took it upon myself to ensure everyone was happy. If someone was upset, I felt responsible. I would replay conversations over and over in my head, picking apart every word I had said, wondering if I needed to apologize or explain myself. It wasn't just an occasional worry—this would absolutely consume me for days afterwards.

As I got older, that feeling of responsibility for the emotions of others didn't go away. When I opened my first gym, I poured everything I had into making sure my members felt valued and cared for. I wanted their time at the gym to be the best part of their day.

That's a great goal, but behind the scenes, I was still playing the same exhausting game—revisiting every interaction and decision, wondering if I could have done more or better. The weight of it was almost debilitating.

Eventually, I hit a breaking point. I realized that I had been tying my sense of worth to how much I could give to others, how much I could achieve, and whether or not people approved of me. But self-worth isn't something that can be earned. It's something you must claim. I had to come to terms with the fact that I was worthy of love, care, and respect—not because of *what I did*, but because of *who I am*. And I am more than enough.

This shift in perspective wasn't instant. It was built through small, intentional actions—setting boundaries, prioritizing my mental and physical health, and learning to let go of the constant need for external validation. Little by little, I began to live by my own standards rather than the expectations I thought others had for me. I stopped chasing approval and started embracing the truth that I was already enough. As my self-worth grew, so did my confidence and resilience. I developed an ability to show up for myself in ways that truly mattered.

Nothing in this book, or in my SHIFTS Framework, will be effective for you if you don't first start by recognizing and reinforcing your self-worth.

Why?

Self-worth is the foundation for everything else.

Without it, the healthiest habits, the best fitness plan, and even the most supportive environment won't create lasting change in your life. But when you believe you are worthy of taking care of yourself, everything shifts. You stop viewing fitness, nutrition, and wellness as obligations and start seeing them as acts of self-love. That's when real transformation begins.

Before we move on, I want to differentiate between self-worth and self-confidence. Both are important, but they're often used interchangeably, yet they're distinctly different.

SELF-WORTH VS. SELF-CONFIDENCE

It's easy to confuse self-worth with self-confidence, but they are not the same thing. Self-worth is the deep-rooted belief that you are inherently valuable and deserving of love, care, and respect—no matter what. It isn't tied to your achievements or your physical appearance. It's not related to whether you have the approval of others. It is stable and unconditional.

You are enough.

Self-confidence, on the other hand, is your belief in your abilities. It fluctuates depending on circumstances—how prepared you feel, how much experience you have, or how others perceive your performance. While self-confidence is important, it is not the foundation of your well-being. Self-worth, however, *is*.

In Jamie Kern Lima's book, *Worthy: How to Believe You Are Enough and Transform Your Life*, she compares self-worth to the foundation of a house and self-confidence to the structure built on top of it. If the foundation is weak, the house won't stand for long.

You might feel confident in some areas of your life—maybe you're great at your job, or you feel strong in your workouts—but without self-worth, those external achievements will never feel like enough. You'll always be chasing the next thing, hoping it will finally make you feel whole.

That's why self-worth has to come *first*. When you have an unshakable sense of self-worth, confidence naturally follows. You know you are enough—not because of what you do, but because of who you are. That's important because you can't always count on others to validate or support you. What happens if or when that support isn't there? You'll need to trust in your own strength to keep going. This was something I definitely learned the hard way.

But when the people closest to you who should be your biggest cheerleaders and supporters let you down, it's definitely challenging to overcome. As a single mom with a young daughter, I heard a lot of criticisms like this from some of the people closest to me:

"You can't be an entrepreneur AND single mom and still live safely and responsibly."

"You're doing fitness and swimwear photoshoots as a single mom and business owner? You must only care about your appearance. How narcissistic!"

"You can't be a professional dancer and cheerleader as a single mom. Those aren't real jobs, and you're being irresponsible. Get a desk job."

"Once you're a mom, you need to give up all the fitness and nutrition stuff."

Even though my daughter and I were thriving and building a life rooted in joy, purpose, independence, and connection, there were still those who questioned and criticized my choices. Never encouraging, always doubting. I had created a way to support us financially, doing what I had dreamed of since I was a little girl. Although our life may have seemed unconventional from the outside, it was rich with meaning and deeply fulfilling.

My daughter grew up surrounded by nature and community, at the beach and in the water. We went camping and hiking and spent time with family and friends. I was able to enroll her in an amazing school, all made possible through my career in fitness and wellness. I was present for her life, her activities, school events, and playdates. And yet, for some, this still wasn't enough. They chose not to see it. But I did, and so did she.

I have loved every single minute of being her mom—even through the tough stuff. She'll always hold a special place in my heart as the one who taught me how to love, lead, and grow. Now, with my son and my partner in our lives, my heart has only grown bigger. They each hold their own unique and deeply cherished place in my life. I dreamed of being my daughter's and my son's mom since I was a little girl creating scrapbooks and making things for my unborn children when I was in elementary school.

As a mom, I've always had, and still have, big goals and dreams, especially when it comes to how I show up for my daughter. Above all, I want her to know without a doubt that she is deeply and unconditionally loved. It has always mattered to me that she feels she can come to me for anything, anytime. I remain passionate and committed to leading by example for her, living a strong, healthy, joy-filled life through simple, mindful choices. I believe that being a steady, loving presence in her life will help her continue to build and grow her own self-worth and give her the courage to go after what she wants.

And speaking of dreams, sometimes we learn our biggest lessons in self-worth while pursuing our own dreams.

LESSONS LEARNED FROM DYNAMIS CROSSFIT

I always knew I wanted to open my own gym. Since I was 8 years old, that dream lived inside me, and when it finally became a reality with Dynamis CrossFit, it was nothing short of surreal. There I was, surrounded by world-class coaches, including a four-time head strength and conditioning coach for the US Bobsled Team and CrossFit Games competitors. These were people at the top of their field, and they wanted to be part of what I was building. It was super wild, amazing, and incredible.

Dynamis CrossFit wasn't just a gym—it was a hub of energy, passion, and innovation. My business partners each brought unique strengths: one owned a fitness equipment company, which meant our gym doubled as a showroom for their latest gear, and the other ran an underground CrossFit apparel company, and a website and marketing company. The name Dynamis itself symbolized divine power, miraculous strength, and potential and inner force.

Why did we choose the name Dynamis? The word "dynamis" is often used to describe the inherent potential energy or capacity to become or act. It's the force or power within someone—not yet fully realized, but always present. It's the seed of action, growth, and transformation. It's the creative, life-giving force within us and our personal power to manifest, act, evolve, and affect the world. In short, Dynamis was an embodiment of what my partners and I were creating together.

Building and growing a gym was everything I had ever wanted. I was living my dream, coaching others, growing an incredible community, and making a tangible impact on people's lives. But as much as the community was growing and the business was thriving, it became clear that parts of my personal life weren't aligned. I was in a relationship with one of my business partners, and when the personal and professional blurred, so did the boundaries.

My life was full. I was living my purpose. I have always thrived and performed well under pressure, and I was boldly leading from the front. As a co-founder, owner, head coach, and gym manager of one of the fastest growing CrossFit gyms in North County—maybe even all of San Diego—I poured myself into building something I believed in. On top of that, I traveled monthly teaching CrossFit Gymnastics Trainer Seminars across the country and the world. In the same breath, I was committed to my own training, my private training clients, running my business, and staying fully present for my daughter and family with school drop-offs and pickups, quality family time, and my daughter's school functions and extracurricular activities.

It was a demanding time, but it was also a very fun life. Beneath the surface, however, I was facing anxiety, imposter syndrome, and the ongoing struggle to prove my worth—to my business partner, to my gym members, and most importantly, to myself. Communication broke down, and it started impacting more than just me. One of the hardest aspects of this trying time was knowing my daughter was watching. I wanted her to see a healthy, strong example of resilience and self-respect. I knew I had a bigger role to play, as a mother and as a leader in my own life. Honoring this truth and choosing what was best for my daughter and me was far from easy, but it was necessary as I moved forward with courage and clarity.

During this time, I sought therapy for my anxiety, and I took my daughter to therapy on a weekly basis as well. My daughter and I made it a priority to remain both mentally and physically healthy by staying active. We played sports, went to the gym, ran, hiked, and spent time at the beach. I wanted her to see me navigating adversity and facing challenges while staying true and authentic to who I am, yet there were moments I felt I was falling short of the high standards I held for myself. I was giving so much to others, but not always standing up for my own worth in personal relationships. And that was hard for me to admit.

I refuse to live in fear, self-doubt, or intimidation, especially when it comes to my purpose. I follow my heart, and I'm fearless in protecting and supporting those I love. I have dedicated my life to helping people live their strongest, healthiest, happiest lives which is why I think I felt so much shame in my struggle (with anxiety) during this time—as a business owner, yes, but even more so as a mom.

In this season of my life, I faced unexpected challenges that shook the foundation of everything I had worked so hard to build, personally and professionally. While it tested me mentally, emotionally, and financially, it also became a powerful turning point.

In the end, I made the decision to step away—not from the business itself, but from the relationship and the day-to-day environment I had once poured so much of myself into. I entrusted the business to my partners and chose to create space for healing, clarity, and alignment. It wasn't a decision made lightly. I had poured so much of my heart into that chapter, but I knew I couldn't keep showing up for everyone else while abandoning myself. At the time, it felt like I was letting go of something I had built with my whole heart and soul.

Today, I see it differently. I see the decision I made as one for survival. I see it as a choice that required an inner strength I didn't know I had at the time.

Looking back, I honor the courage it took to make that decision. I know in my bones it was the best choice I could have made for myself and my daughter in that season of our lives. Yet if I were faced with the same situation today, I wouldn't walk away. Not because it would hurt any less or be any easier, but because the self-worth, confidence, and clarity I have gained since then would allow me to stand my ground differently.

Today, I know how to protect what I've built without abandoning myself in the process.

That experience was painful, but it also became a massive part of my growth and transformation. It taught me what self-worth really means. It showed me that being strong isn't about always pushing through. Sometimes, real strength is knowing when to rest, when to set boundaries, and when to choose yourself, even when it breaks your heart.

And maybe most importantly, it reminded me that I'm allowed to take up space. I'm allowed to protect what matters to me. And I'm absolutely allowed to fight for the life I want and deserve. In hindsight, I see how much I've grown. I see how those experiences shaped me, how they pushed me to recognize my worth and hold stronger boundaries. I've learned how to navigate tough relationships, how to handle confrontation, and communicate in ways that ensure I am heard and respected. More than anything, I've learned to trust myself, my intuition, my instincts, and the quiet knowing that's always been there.

HOW SELF-WORTH AFFECTS FITNESS AND WELLNESS

So what does self-worth have to do with fitness and wellness?

Well, ummm…just about everything!

Fitness and wellness are expressions of self-worth, not just habits to check off a list. When you see yourself as worthy of care and respect, you start making choices that support your well-being—not because you "have to," but because you deserve to.

People often approach fitness from a place of self-criticism, thinking, *I need to lose weight because I don't like how I look* or *I have to work out to make up for what I ate yesterday.* Those mindsets place fitness and nutrition in the category of punishment rather than self-care.

But when you cultivate self-worth, your focus shifts. You move because it makes you feel strong. You fuel your body with good food because you deserve nourishment. You rest because you know your body is valuable and needs recovery. Each of the six SHIFTS becomes a tool to help you reinforce your self-worth.

When you believe you are worthy of love, everything shifts. You no longer view fitness as a temporary fix for an external goal. You see it as a lifelong commitment to treating yourself well. And that's when a lifelong approach to fitness and wellness becomes something that's attainable and sustainable.

The SHIFTS Framework is all about making the little daily decisions to do what's best for your overall fitness and well-being. This isn't you being selfish. This is you saying, "I only get one life, and I want the quality of life I experience to be the best it can be so I can be the best me for me—but also for the people I love that mean the most to me."

That's pretty UNselfish if you ask me.

Just like life is lived a day at a time, your choices will either bring you closer to lifelong fitness and wellness or carry you further away. Your self-worth is the vehicle to drive you closer.

UNCOVERING YOUR SHINE

If self-worth is something you've struggled with, know that you're not alone. We've all been there at times. But you *can* grow your self-worth when you invest some time and energy into it. There are good things inside you, and you're worth the effort it takes to reveal that beauty within.

When I turned 16, my dad gave me an old truck under the condition that I learn how to drive and maintain it. It wasn't much to look at—a 1991 Toyota 4x4 pickup—and it had seen better days. It was a bit of a shop project that all the guys wanted to be part of. My Uncle Fishhead rebuilt the transmission. My dad salvaged some massive mud tires from a super cool Jeep out back. One of the other guys at the shop had a lift kit and wanted a truck to put it on, and mine was the perfect fit for it. With the lift, I practically needed a ladder to get in and out of it. It had dull red paint and years of wear, and there was nothing particularly remarkable about it, but I loved that truck just the way it was and was proud to drive it around.

One day, my neighbor, who ran a detailing and pinstriping business, told me something interesting. He said if I was willing to put in some work and elbow grease, there was a way to restore the paint to its original shine. No expensive repaint, no shortcuts—just a chemical compound and some serious elbow grease. He agreed to show me how and provide the materials and tools I'd need, so I decided to go for it.

Now keep in mind that it was the middle of a hot, sticky Houston summer. We're talking upper 90s and high humidity, but I didn't care. I got up early and got to work polishing it inch by inch, rubbing away years of grime and build-up with good old muscle magic. It took two full days, from sunup to sundown, but when I was finished, my truck looked brand new. I couldn't wait to show my dad! When I drove up to his auto shop, he didn't even recognize the truck! He even thought I had taken it in for a professional paint job.

But I hadn't—I had simply uncovered what was already there.

That truck's transformation reminds me of the self-worth journey many of us are on. Just like that beautiful paint job was hidden under layers of grime, our confidence, strength, and resilience are often buried under self-doubt, neglect, and years of conditioning that tell us we're not enough. I know that's what I experienced.

I could have taken the easy route with my truck. I could have paid for a new paint job and had someone else do it, but I'm so glad I didn't. I'm thrilled that I put in the time and effort to uncover its original shine because otherwise, I'd have never experienced the pride I felt in the hard work I put in.

The same goes for our fitness and wellness. Quick fixes—like crash diets or medications—might seem like the answers, but they don't address what's underneath.

True transformation happens when you commit to the process, work through the hard stuff, and allow the best version of yourself to shine through.

Your worth is already there. It just takes consistency, effort, and self-love to reveal it. That's where vision comes in. When you start showing up for yourself with consistency and care, you're not only affirming your worth—you're also shaping who you're becoming. Growth doesn't happen by accident. It happens when you get clear on who you want to be and start taking aligned action toward that future version of you.

THE AVATAR EXERCISE

When you think about building your self-worth, you're not just doing it for who you are today. You're also doing it for who you will become tomorrow. So let's first figure out who you want to become, then create a plan to grow into that version of you.

Growing up in gymnastics, my coaches would have us lie down on the floor with our eyes closed and visualize ourselves doing our routines top to bottom perfectly for weeks before a competition. In my mind's eye, I went over every detail, and when I say every detail, I mean every detail. It sounds like it would be easy, but it was actually pretty hard to do. It was worth it though, because once I had that detailed visual, it became part of me, and I was able to complete my routine much more precisely and confidently. I realized I had everything I needed inside me to get the result I wanted. I just had to visualize, then do what that visualized version of me would do.

It wasn't until years later that I realized I could apply this same principle to more than just physical feats. Last year I took a workshop by Wendy Porter of Crowned for Success. In it, she taught all attendees how to build our own avatars as a way of visualizing who we wanted to be and how we could use those visualizations to grow our self-worth. We sat down with a journal and got specific about who the ultimate version of ourselves is, right down to the last detail. You'll have a chance to do the version I've created of this exercise for yourself a little later in this chapter. For now, here are some of the questions and answers I recorded for my avatar:

What does my avatar drive? I drive a hybrid BMW SUV—white with leather interior—all-wheel drive.

Where does my avatar live? I live at my NZ Fitness and Wellness Ranch and Retreat Center. It's over ten acres with a full-sized barn gym, recovery center, yoga studio, vineyard, and lake. It also has a fruit and vegetable farm, a chicken coop, goats, a cow, and horses. I'll offer tiny home rentals and Airbnb to responsible amazing guests and tenants plus CrossFit classes, private training, and retreats.

How much money does my avatar have in savings and investments? I desire to live debt-free with an abundance of passive monthly income I can save, invest, and use to continue to grow my business ventures and real estate business—and also help causes and people I truly believe in.

How does my avatar behave? I behave with class, grace, boldness, authenticity, soulfulness, passion, strength, energy, vivaciousness, vitality, grit, resilience, and honesty.

How does my avatar dress? I dress well—super classy, modern, fit.

My hair is always done—whether that is up, down, or doing its own thing, ha ha.

Where does my avatar travel? I travel the world! Road trips to all the national parks, US coastlines, and tropical islands. I also travel across Europe and beyond!

I couldn't believe how much clarity this exercise gave me!

Once I finished writing everything down, I took a deeper look and asked myself some tough questions, like:

If this is who I'm striving to be, does my life show it?

Are my actions, thoughts, and decisions taking me closer or further from that version of me?

Those are some pretty straightforward questions, aren't they? I encourage you to ask yourself these questions too, and be honest with your answers. No one will see them but you. Now that I have a clear vision of who my avatar is, those two questions have become my guideline for how I show up as my ideal self every day.

I did that exercise a year ago, but I already see the results of it in my life. Here are some things I have achieved since doing the avatar exercise.

What kind of car do I drive? I paid off and sold my Ford C-Max Hybrid, and I now drive a BMW AWD SUV. (Side note: When you have a basic understanding of vehicle maintenance, maintaining a foreign luxury vehicle doesn't have to be expensive.)

How much money do I have in savings and investments?

I am now debt free, and I am saving more than I ever have in my entire life each month. I am making some big progress on investing monthly and seeing tons of growth and solid returns on my investments.

How do I behave? I can say I behave with class, grace, boldness, authenticity, soulfulness, passion, strength, energy, vivaciousness, vitality, grit, resilience, and honesty on a consistent basis.

How do I dress? I dress well—super classy, modern, fit. My hair is always done…whether that is up, down, or doing its own thing, ha ha.

Where do I travel? I took the leap and am going on my first ever yoga retreat on a little island off the coast of Greece later this spring and adding some gallivanting around Italy to this trip! I've already done some traveling this year to Las Vegas for a fitness conference and with my family to Texas. My family and I will be traveling to Dallas and then the Hill Country (Canyon Lake, New Braunfels, Gruene, the Guadalupe River, etc.) and Siesta Key, Florida this summer and fall. We also have several camping trips in the works throughout California and surrounding areas.

Now, I'm still working on my fitness and wellness ranch and wine vineyard. I've been talking with a loan officer, my bookkeeper, my accountant, my business coach, and several real estate agents about this project currently. It feels like I have so far to go before this becomes a reality, but I'm doing what I can now to continue moving the needle in that direction.

Okay, now it's your turn!

Head to the Book Resources page of my website. Inside, you'll find a "Create Your Avatar" downloadable PDF that you can print and fill out. I also included my own detailed version of my answers to this exercise to help give you a bit of inspiration and jog your creativity. Check the Resources section at the end of this book for the link to my Book Resources page.

Filling out the "Create Your Avatar" sheet is a great way to evaluate your self-worth because you can use it to take inventory of your life to determine what's working and what's not. The best way to do this is to take a week or so and track your day-to-day behaviors and habits as you are right now. Then look at your behaviors and habits through the lens of your avatar. Are your actions, thoughts, and decisions bringing you closer or further away from the ultimate you? Later, I'll show you a concrete way to do this with the help of a free downloadable SHIFTS tracker in chapter 10.

MAKING ADJUSTMENTS THAT LAST

Today, I measure my decisions by my avatar. I consider the standards I've set for myself and ask, "Will this choice help me become more or less like the best version of myself?" As long as I do this, I can anchor myself in the foundations of the life I want to maintain and the person I want to be, even in dark, lonely times that don't make sense. My avatar is my plumb line, even right down to what I eat, how I move, what I listen to, and what I watch.

As you look at your habits and behaviors, you'll find areas in your life that need adjusting in order to help you become the best version of yourself.

Congratulations—that means you're one step closer to leveling up! This is a lifelong journey, and there's not a single person on the planet who has 100% arrived at perfection overnight (or ever)! True and lasting transformation starts one step at a time. Focus on progress over perfection, and choose one simple adjustment to start making today that will help you get closer to your ideal self.

Instead of massive overnight change, think of your growth in terms of subtractions and additions. When you subtract one unhealthy behavior or habit, add a positive one to balance things out. For example, I did this by swapping TV for music and sugary drinks for water.

Your small actions matter because they're a vote for the type of person you want to become! If you've struggled with self-confidence and self-worth, making these daily choices are so important because they help you shift your beliefs about who you are.

Jim Kwik, brain coach and author of the book *Limitless: Upgrade Your Brain, Learn Anything Faster, and Unlock Your Exceptional Life*, talks about how choices are the key to change: "If you want to create a new result in your life, which most of us do, you have to make a new choice. There are only four fundamental ways to make a change. You either could stop something, you could start something, you could do less of something, or you could do more of something. That is literally it."[1]

As humans, we tend to make this harder than it is, but personal growth and transformation are the results of small, daily choices you make to add behaviors that are healthy and remove those that are unhealthy, one at a time. Lifelong fitness and wellness are the same—they're the result of making small shifts in your sleep, hydration, nutrition, movement, and mindset over time. When you start building up your self-worth, one choice at a time, that's when you start to grow into the best version of you.

KEY TAKEAWAYS FOR CHAPTER 4

1. **Self-worth ≠ self-confidence.** Confidence is about what you can do. Worth is about who you are—and you don't have to earn it.
2. **Adversity teaches.** Hard seasons, like when I stepped away from Dynamis CrossFit, can help you learn to set boundaries and trust your worth.
3. **Worth fuels healthy choices.** When you believe you're worthy, you move, eat, and rest out of self-love, not punishment.
4. **Uncover your shine.** Like buffing out an old truck, revealing your worth takes work, but the beauty is already there.
5. **Visualize your future self.** Use the avatar exercise to guide daily choices that align with who you're becoming.
6. **Change is built, not forced.** Small, consistent shifts led by self-worth create lasting progress. And progress will always win over "perfection", because perfection isn't actually attainable.

[1] Jim Kwik, *Limitless*. (Carlsbad, CA: Hay House, 2020).
These quotes are provided via fair use for educational purposes to verify my teachings.

Chapter 5

Consistency

Have you ever seen one of those ten-day fitness challenges advertised online? They make big, flashy promises like "lose ten pounds in ten days." People get all fired up, and for ten days they change their diet, their sleep schedule, their reading habits, and their workout routine—all at once. Maybe they make it through the ten days, but it's a LOT. The minute the challenge is over, they fall off and go nuts on all the things they couldn't do or eat during the challenge.

This can lead to them beating themselves up for not sticking with the program. Sometimes it leads to a shame spiral where they decide they'll never change. It can even cause depression. So much change was packed into such a short amount of time, there was no opportunity to build healthy, sustainable habits that could last. This type of all-or-nothing approach sets people up to fail, and that's NOT what I mean when I talk about consistency.

We're in this for the long haul, right? Fitness and wellness are worth so much more than a ten-day challenge, and that means our approach to consistency needs to be achievable for anyone regardless of age, weight, gender, or ability.

Before we dive into my SHIFTS Framework in Part 2 of this book, it's important to keep in mind that fitness and wellness are created one action step and one healthy choice at a time. As you take action steps and make healthy choices part of your daily life over time, you will see results. The good news is, you can build consistency as you go, you don't have to tackle consistency in every single piece of the framework all at once.

CONSISTENCY THE SUSTAINABLE WAY

For sustainable transformation and long-term health and wellness benefits, you need to start at the beginning and build a strong foundation for fitness and wellness, brick by brick. Little actions performed consistently over time add up to really BIG things. The goals you're pursuing won't happen all at once, and that's okay.

Think about what happens when you learn a new skill— like when you learned how to drive a car. You weren't an expert at it right away. Your parents or driver's ed teacher probably sprouted a few gray hairs teaching you. But day after day you showed up, put yourself in the driver's seat, turned the key, and practiced. Because you knew the ability to drive was going to be an important one for you to have for the rest of your life. All that practice helped you become the confident driver you are today.

Your fitness and wellness are going to be important to you for the rest of your life too, so it's worth taking a mindful approach. This will make it a lot easier to continue to show up for yourself even when you don't *feel* like training, eating healthy, or going to bed at a decent hour.

And I'm right there too—some days I get to the gym and I'm tired. I have a toddler at home, and I don't always bounce out of my nice, comfortable bed like the Energizer Bunny. Welcome to reality, right? But you know what? I can feel tired and still choose consistency. Maybe in order to give myself grace, my workout won't look like I originally planned. I can modify my training session when I've had a rough night with little sleep, which is better than skipping it completely.

When you stay consistent in the small changes you're making, even when you don't feel like showing up, you build *consistency muscles* that will benefit you for a lifetime. Now, of course, if you're sick or there's something else outside of your control that interrupts your daily health habits, that's legitimate. Sometimes showing up for yourself is dealing with that family emergency or staying home in bed to rest and recover. But as soon as you're able, get right back to it with self-love—the same love you would give your significant other or your children.

PRACTICAL CONSISTENCY-BUILDING TIPS

Building sustainable fitness habits doesn't have to be complicated, and when you've built discipline through consistency, you don't have to rely on willpower. Over the years, I've learned some practical tools and strategies that can help you stay on track and make fitness a natural and enjoyable part of your life. In this section, I'll walk you through each strategy one at a time.

Schedule Your Workouts Like Appointments

One of the best pieces of advice I can give is to treat each training session like you would any other important appointment. Put them on your calendar, set reminders, and protect that time. Think of it as a nonnegotiable "fitness date" with yourself. It doesn't matter if it's 20 minutes or an hour. What matters is that you've carved out time to move your body.

When you schedule your sessions in advance, it removes the decision-making process. You don't have to think about if or when you're going to work out because it's already planned and decided. And when life inevitably gets busy, you're less likely to skip your session because it's already built into your day.

Start Small and Build Over Time

Fitness is a marathon, not a sprint. If you're just starting out, don't feel like you have to jump straight into a six-day training plan. Start with two or three workouts a week and focus on being consistent. Once you've built the habit and it feels like a natural part of your routine, you can gradually add more.

In chapter 11, you'll learn some simple bodyweight movements. In the Resources section of this book, you can access my free 7-day training program and download the appendix to this book, which features even more bodyweight movements with step-by-step photos and video demonstrations. If you're brand new to exercise, you could start there. Stick with that for a few weeks, and when you're ready, add an extra session or increase the intensity of your workouts. The goal is to build a habit that is sustainable, not overwhelming.

Plan Ahead to Remove Barriers

We all have those days when working out feels like the last thing we want to do. That's why planning ahead is so important. Lay out your workout clothes the night before, have your water bottle ready, your meals (aka your fuel) prepped, and know exactly what workout you're going to do. These simple actions remove the mental friction that can make it easy to skip your session. If you're working out at home, create a dedicated space for it. If you're going to the gym, pack your bag the night before. The fewer obstacles you have to overcome, the easier it will be to stay consistent.

Focus on What You *Can* Do

Fitness is about progress, not perfection. There will be days when you're tired, stressed, or short on time and that's okay. On those days, focus on what you can do, even if it's only ten minutes of movement. A quick walk, some light stretching, or a few rounds of bodyweight exercises can still make a big difference. The point is to keep the habit alive, even if it's not your most intense or structured workout. Something is always better than nothing, and those small efforts add up over time.

Celebrate Small Wins

One of the most powerful ways to stay motivated is to celebrate your progress along the way. It doesn't have to be a big milestone. Maybe you did one more push-up than last week, lifted a little heavier, or simply showed up for every workout you planned. Take a moment to acknowledge those victories, because they matter. Celebrating small wins reinforces the habit of you showing up for yourself in this way and helps you stay connected to your progress. It's a reminder that every step forward is a step closer to your goals.

Mix It Up to Keep It Fun

If you're getting bored with your workouts, you're less likely to stick with them. That's why variety is so important. Try different types of movement, and incorporate things like strength training, yoga, cycling, hiking, swimming, or even dancing on your active recovery days. Explore new environments, like outdoor workouts or group classes, to keep things fresh and exciting. Mixing it up also challenges your body in new ways and helps you build well-rounded fitness. So don't be afraid to experiment and find what lights you up.

Find Accountability and Support

Having someone to keep you accountable can make all the difference. This could be a coach, a workout buddy, or even a community of like-minded people. When you know someone else is counting on you, you're more likely to show up.

If you can, work with a coach or trainer who can guide you and structure your training and programming to your goals. They'll not only provide accountability, but also make sure your training is effective and safe. And if a trainer isn't in your budget, find a friend or group to keep you motivated: Ask them to encourage you to stay consistent.

Prioritize Recovery

Recovery is just as important as the workout itself. Make sure you're giving your body the time it needs to rest and repair. This includes things like:

- **Hydration:** Drink plenty of water to support your muscles and joints. (See Section 7.2 for specific recommendations on hydration.)
- **Protein:** Fuel your body with enough protein to aid recovery and build strength. (See Section 7.3 for specific recommendations on protein.)
- **Sleep:** Aim for quality sleep, as it's crucial for recovery and overall performance. (See Section 7.1 for specific recommendations on sleep.)

Active recovery days, where you add in stretching, yoga, or a leisurely walk, can also help you stay consistent while giving your body a break from intense training.

Be Patient and Kind to Yourself

Finally, give yourself grace.

Building sustainable fitness habits takes time, and it's normal to have ups and downs along the way. What matters most is that you keep showing up for yourself, even when it feels hard. Fitness isn't about being perfect. It's about progress, consistency, and building a life that supports your goals and enables you to live a high-quality life. And wellness means finding balance when it comes to your nutrition and recovery—plus finding a consistent groove for your fitness.

When you focus on these practical tools, fitness stops feeling like a chore and starts becoming a natural part of your lifestyle. Remember, it's not about doing everything perfectly—it's about doing what you can, showing up for yourself consistently, and finding joy in the process.

You've got this!

ADDITIONS AND SUBTRACTIONS

We're all busy, and sometimes the thought of changing your lifestyle seems overwhelming and impossible. If change is hard for you or the word consistency gives you hives, try this trick I show my clients. Instead of thinking about your fitness and wellness as having to make a bunch of changes, think about them in terms of making additions and subtractions.

If you're adding something new to your life, what can you leave behind in order to make room for something new that will benefit you? Or, if you're removing something from your life, what can you add to fill the gap? Here are a few ideas of additions and subtractions to get your creativity flowing.

Swap a Sweet for Protein

Let's say you know you need to eat more protein. Instead of completely changing your entire diet overnight, make a swap. Switch out a sugary snack like a candy bar with one that's healthier with more grams of protein, like berries and plain Greek yogurt or a whole food protein bar like a Rise Bar. That's more manageable, especially in the beginning. Over time, make more swaps until you're consuming the optimal amount of protein for you.

Replace a Cup of Coffee with a Glass of Water

Need to drink more water? Swap out a cup of coffee or soda for a glass of water daily. When I was in high school, I stopped drinking beverages with sugar in them. I knew the sugar wasn't doing me any favors, so I drank water instead. It was a super simple swap, but within weeks I noticed a pretty big change in body composition and overall energy.

Trade TV for an Extra Hour of Sleep

Need more sleep? Maybe try turning off the TV or other screens an hour earlier to allow your brain to wind down sooner.

Additions and subtractions are simple, consistent changes that are extremely doable.

When you make additions and subtractions, it helps keep things balanced, and a balanced life is more manageable. When you practice consistency in the small things, you build new lifestyle habits gradually over time, making you more likely to stay on track while moving in the direction you want to go. Now that you know what these strategies are in more detail, let's take a step back and take a look at what they mean collectively when we're building those consistency muscles.

Here's a simple thing you can do for yourself that will help you reshape your mindset as you build consistency.

AFFIRMATIONS FOR CONSISTENCY

Do you struggle to believe you're capable of being consistent? Affirmations, or positive statements that reinforce a belief, mindset, or the outcome you want, can be super powerful.

Affirmations can help you grow your confidence while you focus on the outcomes you want. Repeating affirmations consistently can also help reshape your mindset.

Whenever I want to shift my mindset or raise my energy, I use affirmations to help me rewire my thought patterns, refocus my energy, reprogram my limiting beliefs, and align my thinking with the version of myself I am becoming. I find an affirmation that helps and repeat it anywhere from 5 to 25 times, 6 to 7 days a week for several months.

Here are some examples of good ones to get you started:

- "I am worthy. I am enough."
- "I am consistent. I show up for myself daily."
- "I am capable of achieving my goals."
- "I trust my body and its ability to grow stronger every day."
- "I am strong. I am brave. I am confident."
- "I embody success. I create my own reality, and I trust myself."

Remember that even a small step is still a step. Building longevity and a high-quality life will benefit you for a lifetime. It makes sense that it takes a lifetime to build up to that a little bit at a time.

Be patient. BUT take action and do what you can now.

Give yourself grace.

Stay accountable to yourself by also being accountable to someone else who you respect.

Find ways to show up every day as your ideal YOU.

And be sure to celebrate your progress every step of the way!

KEY TAKEAWAYS FOR CHAPTER 5

1. **Consistency isn't all-or-nothing.** Real progress comes from small, steady steps, not trying to do everything at once. Think lifestyle, not quick fix.
2. **Make it fit your life.** Wellness shouldn't feel like punishment. Show up, practice, and build over time.
3. **Simple = sustainable.** Prep ahead. Start small. Modify when needed. Progress is about showing up, not going hard.
4. **Small swaps matter.** Trade soda for water, scrolling for sleep, candy for protein. Tiny choices lead to big change.
5. **Speak it until you believe it.** Use affirmations like: "I am consistent. I show up for myself." Your brain listens, so give it something worth repeating.

PART 2

Live STRONG, Live HEALTHY, Live HAPPY

Chapter 6
Shifting Gears

My dad and I had just left the DMV and my brand new learner's permit was in my pocket. As we approached the vehicle we'd driven—a standard 1991 Toyota 4x4 pickup my dad had been working on in his auto shop—he tossed me the keys.

"Do you want to drive now that you have your permit?"

"Umm, okay," I said. I climbed into the cab and scooted the seat up as far as it would go so my foot could push the clutch all the way to the floor. Gripping the wheel so tightly my knuckles turned white, I managed to pull out of the parking lot and make it to the first stoplight. My dad was in the passenger seat, calm as ever, completely unfazed.

We sat there, the first car in line to turn left to get onto the feeder road that merged onto the freeway, the light turned green. I took a deep breath, slowly lifted my foot off the clutch, and—stalled. The truck jerked forward, then stopped.

Behind us, there was honking. So much honking. The light was still green, so I frantically tried again. I pressed the clutch, moved into first gear, slowly released, and—stalled. Again.

More honking. Frustrated drivers started whipping around us, throwing their hands up in the air. My heart pounded, and my eyes started to sting with tears. I wanted to quit, to unbuckle my seatbelt, slide over to the passenger seat, and ask my dad to drive us home. But when I turned to look at him, expecting him to be frustrated or impatient, he wasn't.

"They're fine," he said, nodding toward the impatient drivers. "Let them go around. We'll get through it."

I nodded, took a shaky breath, and tried again. This time, the car lurched forward just as the light turned yellow. I barely made it through the intersection before it switched to red behind me, but I did it! We were moving! But then, panic hit me again.

I was getting on the freeway...and I was only in first gear!

To be honest, I had no intention of shifting. I was barely holding it together as it was. I decided I would rather ride in first gear all the way home than risk another stall. Dad, however, had other ideas. In that same steady, even voice, he simply said, "Okay, now I need you to push the clutch in. I'll shift gears for you."

I hesitated but followed his instructions. I pressed the clutch, he shifted, and we were moving—smoothly. By the time we made it home, I had sweat through my shirt. (Did I mention this was Texas in the summertime and the truck's AC had gone out on the way to the DMV?) But Dad had helped me through the hardest part, and I was on my way.

SHIFTING GEARS IN DRIVING AND IN LIFE

That day has stuck with me for so many reasons. Yes, I learned how to drive a stick shift (eventually), but more than that, I learned a lesson that would carry over into so many areas of my life: The only way forward is through.

When something feels scary, uncomfortable, or overwhelming, we instinctively want to avoid it. We tell ourselves we're not ready, that whatever we're trying to do is too hard, that maybe there's an easier way. But avoiding the thing we *need* to do doesn't get us anywhere—it keeps us stuck.

I could have easily given up that day. I could have decided I wasn't cut out for a manual transmission. In fact, I called my dad later that day and asked him if they could switch out the standard transmission for an automatic so I'd never have to go through that kind of experience again. Haha!

Of course, that wouldn't have helped me grow. He convinced me to keep trying. And you know what? There were times I stalled. There were times I struggled. But eventually? I figured out how to keep moving forward.

The same is true in fitness and wellness, and in life.

How many times do we tell ourselves *I'll start when I'm ready*? Or *I'll make a change when things slow down*? Or *I just need everything to be perfect first*? The truth is, there is never a perfect time to start.

At some point, you just have to decide to start where you're at, even if that means you have to scoot the seat way up so your little legs can reach the pedals, press the clutch, shift gears, and go. But what if you already feel stuck where you're at? Then what?

GETTING STUCK IN FIRST GEAR

We've all had those stuck-on-the-freeway-in-first-gear moments. It's easier to stay in first gear. It feels safer. But progress happens when we're willing to shift gears.

When I work with clients, I see this all the time. They'll start their fitness journey full of motivation, ready to go all in. But the moment they hit resistance—whether it's a tough workout, a busy schedule, or self-doubt—they stall. They hesitate to push past that discomfort because it's unfamiliar. It's intimidating.

And I get it—because I've been there. But here's the thing: staying stuck in first gear won't get you to where you want to go. At some point, you have to choose to focus your mindset and trust yourself enough to shift, even when it feels scary. Even when you're not sure if you're doing things right. Even when you're sweating and frustrated and overwhelmed. Because the growth and progress you want is on the other side of that shift.

THROUGH, NOT AROUND

If I had given up that day, I wouldn't have learned how to drive that truck. And if I hadn't driven that truck, I wouldn't have built the confidence that came with mastering something difficult. That's how life works. The only way to overcome a challenge is to go through it. There's no shortcut. No way around. No magic trick that makes it easy. But there is something that makes it *possible*. The willingness to take action anyway.

When you decide to push the clutch, shift the gear, and keep going—even when it feels messy, even when you stall, even when you're scared—you can accomplish more than you ever dreamed. Because the more you practice, the better you get. And before you know it, you're cruising—confident, strong, and capable of driving anywhere you want to go. And trust me—once you learn how to shift gears by taking action anyway, you can accomplish anything. But where do you start? With your *brain*.

Henry Ford once said, "Whether you think you can or you think you can't, you're right." I believe this is so true. If you think you can keep going, nothing can stop you. If you don't believe you can, nothing will get you there. Your mind is a powerful tool in your fitness and wellness journey, which is why it's the "T" for "Thoughts" in SHIFTS. We'll go deeper into mindset in Section 7.5. But before we do, I want to give you four simple steps that will help you prep your mindset to get started with SHIFTS.

Challenges will come. We're always bumping up against hurdles in our minds, but we have a choice of how we deal with them. Growing a strong mindset will help you see those hurdles as opportunities instead of obstacles and as fuel instead of failures. If the SHIFTS Framework is the roadmap to your goals, then your mindset is like the compass that helps keep you on the right path! Here are the four steps to strengthening your mindset so you can be ready for whatever comes your way.

Step 1: Become Aware of Your Mindset

Nothing brings up mindset challenges like doing something new. Fifteen years ago, I stepped into a different adventure when I began leading CrossFit classes for adults—and it was more challenging than I expected.

As a coach, it's my job to make sure everyone moves safely and with good technique.

In small group settings, that means helping clients choose the right progression, load, and volume so they can maintain solid form while still hitting the intended goal of each session.

But not everyone appreciates coaching feedback. In my experience, women have been more open and eager to learn. They want clear, step-by-step guidance to make sure they're moving correctly. Many men, especially early in my CrossFit coaching career, were a different story. Some didn't respond to my cues at all. Others cut reps short or sacrificed form in the name of competition—and some outright ignored me, especially in strength training.

That felt discouraging and I questioned whether I was cut out to coach groups. But instead of giving up, I chose awareness. I asked myself: *Where's my mindset right now? How am I doing emotionally, mentally, and physically?* That shift made all the difference.

Today, 99.9% of my experiences coaching men are the opposite of what they were. Because I worked on my mindset, I now experience far more respect and openness from athletes across the board—and the difference is amazing.

Was it fun to check my mindset in that season? No. It was uncomfortable. But facing it head on is what helped me grow. Now, it's your turn. Take a moment to read the following statements and consider where your mindset is today.

SELF-ASSESSMENT: HOW'S MY MINDSET?

Check the statements that apply to you. When you're done, read through the statements you've checked and ask yourself, "Am I choosing to focus my thoughts in a more positive or negative direction?" If they're mostly negative, it's time to work on strengthening your mindset using steps two, three, and four below.

- I often choose to focus on the positive side of things.
- When setbacks happen, my brain immediately jumps to the worst-case scenario.
- I love thinking of fun ways to turn a challenge into an opportunity.
- I talk myself out of trying things I know will be difficult.
- I don't mind being challenged because I know it means I'll grow.
- If something doesn't come easy, I often stop or want to stop.

What did you uncover? When it comes to mindset, we all have areas that can be improved. None of us are perfect, but the good news is, there's no limit to the level of growth our mindsets can achieve. And we're going to talk more about mindset in the next steps.

Step 2: Acknowledge Each Thought

One of the first thoughts that popped up for me when teaching group fitness classes was, "Man, teaching kids is a breeze compared to coaching adults!" I was tempted to shove the thought to the back of my mind so I wouldn't have to deal with it. I wanted to love coaching adults, not feel stressed about it, but I knew pretending everything was fine wasn't going to help. Instead, I acknowledged that I didn't like how things were going.

Once you're aware of where you want your mindset to be, it's easier to identify when you need to shift the way you think. When you catch yourself, call it out. Then ask yourself how you can adjust. *"Okay, this is not where I want to be mentally right now. What can I do about it?"* This is how you can help yourself transition into the next step where you go opportunity hunting.

Step 3: Find the Opportunity

I couldn't control the way some of the guys I coached in small group classes received my coaching feedback, but I knew there had to be an opportunity for growth in the situation somewhere. As I reflected on this, I recognized I could use what I was experiencing to work on my coaching skills so I could become a better coach.

The next step to training your mindset is to identify the opportunity in your current situation. In every obstacle or setback, I believe there's an opportunity to grow and get stronger. And I like to ask myself some questions that help make things more clear. Do you have a situation where you're looking for the opportunity in the middle of a struggle that challenges your mindset? Here are some questions to ask yourself that can help:

What could happen if I change nothing?

What *can* I control in this situation—what or where is there an opportunity?

What are three things I could change or do differently?

What would happen if I made those changes?

As you look at your answers, you'll probably be surprised at how the obstacle shrinks down to size when compared to the opportunity! And this leads us into the next step, which is all about possibility.

Step 4: Get Creative

I knew if I learned how to tactfully address situations I encountered as a coach, clients would become more open to receiving my feedback. This was tough for me. I was a bit more on the quiet and reserved side, and speaking in front of a group definitely pushed me out of my comfort zone. But this was my passion and my calling. I would not allow fear to stop me, so I started approaching these circumstances like a challenge or a game.

I began mentally preparing even more for my classes ahead of time, reading books and learning how to build rapport with clients while standing my ground so they'd be less defensive and more open to receiving coaching feedback. I used learning tools that I knew my brain would find fun. Figuring out how to communicate effectively with each person, depending on their unique needs, was key. That was something I worked hard to learn. It was all about finding ways to overcome my reserved default approach. After working hard and adjusting my approaches, I now feel confident coaching anyone in any environment.

Once you're firmly focused on the opportunity, give yourself permission to get creative. Who says mindset growth can't be fun? Approach whatever hard thing is in front of you, whether it's working with a difficult client, giving up soda, or running a 5K with the attitude of "How can I make this fun?" There's no one right way to meet a goal. You can be creative about how you get there.

It won't all be a walk in the park, but that's a good thing! You may be temporarily uncomfortable. You may be challenged physically and mentally. But when you find ways to make it fun and stick it out, you are developing a wonderful and effective way to grow and strengthen your mindset and mental health, not only for the short term, but for the rest of your life.

In his book, *Limitless: Upgrade Your Brain, Learn Anything Faster, and Unlock Your Exceptional Life*, Jim Kwik talks about how our brains can be changed and shaped by our actions and our environments.[1] That means we're not stuck in the same patterns. We can train our brains to look for opportunities instead of obstacles, and that opens doors. It makes life more fun, more creative, and more fulfilling. Instead of thinking, *I can't do this,* I choose to see challenges as puzzles to solve or fears to face. I've learned that when I approach life with an open mind and a willingness to grow, even the hardest moments can become stepping stones to something greater.

Ultimately, staying consistent with your fitness and wellness goals is about embracing a lifestyle of readiness, both mentally and physically. When you strengthen your body, you prove to yourself that you can do hard things, which strengthens your mindset. When you put in the effort, you're creating a life where you can say yes to new opportunities without hesitation. And to me, that is worth everything!

As you dive into the SHIFTS Framework in the next chapter, I encourage you to stay focused on the fun in the process and the reward at the end. After a tough training session is over, you'll feel the short-term benefits like more energy, a boosted mood, and a sense of accomplishment in the results of your labor. And over time, you'll experience the long-term benefits of stronger muscles, lower body fat composition, increased energy, overall better fitness and wellness, and a higher quality of life.

Want to learn more about your body composition? I love using the body composition app, Spren. Flip to the Resources section of this book to learn how to get access.

KEY TAKEAWAYS FOR CHAPTER 6

1. **Start with mindset.** Motivation fades—action creates confidence. Don't wait to feel ready. Move anyway.
2. **Start where you are.** Forget perfect. Begin small, messy, and real. Growth starts with showing up even before you know how to shift.
3. **Shifting is growth.** Comfort keeps you stuck. Change requires courage and a willingness to try something new.
4. **The only way is through.** You can't avoid the hard stuff—but going through it builds lifelong strength and confidence.
5. **Mindset is your strongest muscle.** Showing up when it's hard builds mental strength and resilience that impacts every part of your life.

---

[1] Jim Kwik, *Limitless: Upgrade Your Brain, Learn Anything Faster, and Unlock Your Exceptional Life.*
Carlsbad, CA: Hay House, 2020.

Chapter 7

The SHIFTS
Framework Revealed

SECTION 7.0: INTRODUCTION TO THE SHIFTS FRAMEWORK

Fitness and wellness are not about fleeting trends. They're about cultivating a lifelong journey of strength, health, and happiness so you can live the life you want long into the future. That's where my SHIFTS Framework comes in. These six principles are the cornerstone of living your strongest, healthiest, and happiest life. They guide you to not only dream about what that life could look like for you, but also teach you how to take practical, sustainable steps to achieve it.

Each element of the SHIFTS Framework represents a foundational aspect of fitness and wellness. Together, they form a holistic system that empowers you to prioritize your well-being while balancing the demands of life. Whether you're a busy parent, a professional with a packed schedule, or someone simply striving to feel stronger and more capable, when you're consistent, this framework will meet you where you are and help you grow.

Here's a sneak peek at what I cover over the course of this chapter:

Section 7.1: Sleep

Section 7.2: Hydration

Section 7.3: Intake (Sustainable Nutrition)

Section 7.4: Fitness

Section 7.5: Thoughts (Mindset)

Section 7.6: Sunshine

Why these six things? Because they work. Through over 38 years of training and competing, and more than 25 years coaching—plus living through my own ups and downs—I've seen these principles transform lives, and not just for my clients, but for mine as well. It literally saved my life. What you need to know, though, is that SHIFTS is about progress, not perfection. You'll learn how to take things step by step and build SHIFTS into your life by making consistent, intentional choices that lead to long-term success.

My story is messy, and it's painful. My life has been far from perfect. It has been filled with heartbreak, but it's also filled with resilience and a fierce desire to live my life on my own terms. I've made it through trauma, single motherhood, rebuilding after losses, and redefining what it means to be strong, happy, and healthy. And that's what I want to share with others. Fitness isn't just about losing weight, being thin, or chasing a quick fix—it's about creating a life where you feel capable, confident, and free. It's about knowing that you have the strength to face whatever comes your way, and that no matter what, you're worth taking care of.

As you move through this chapter, you'll discover how these six shifts can reshape not just your fitness journey, but your entire approach to health and wellness. You'll find practical tips, real-life stories, and actionable strategies to help you create a life filled with energy, purpose, and joy. So… are you ready to make the SHIFT?

SECTION 7.1: SLEEP

The first three weeks of my daughter's life were a blur of pain and delirium. I had a rough delivery and a long, painful recovery from an episiotomy and other physical trauma that resulted from the birthing process. It was so bad I couldn't even sit down, which made breastfeeding a real challenge. And that donut pillow they sent me home with from the hospital was *so* not helpful.

As a first-time mom, I didn't know anything about sleep training or feeding schedules for babies. I kept hearing people say, "Just follow your baby's cues. She'll let you know." But how? I'd feed her and ten minutes later she'd be crying. I was a mess—literally falling asleep propped up trying to feed her in all these weird positions because I was in so much pain.

Three weeks went by and I had barely slept at all. Then my aunt called. She's an amazing woman, and I've always really admired her. She was a competitive athlete growing up and was a teacher for 30 years. She's also an amazing mom to two awesome boys who are now all grown up. When she asked me how I was doing, it all came spilling out.

"I don't know what to do! She's eating like every five minutes! I haven't slept in three weeks, and I don't know how much longer I can go on like this. I can't function." Add in the pain from my episiotomy (which wasn't healing well, probably because I wasn't sleeping), and I was a hot mess.

Immediately, she told me about a book she read that had helped her get her babies on a schedule for sleeping, eating, and waking and mailed me a copy. Desperate for sleep, I was willing to try anything. I'm not saying this will work for everyone, but I read it and started getting my daughter on a schedule to help her settle into eating and sleeping patterns. It really worked for her. She started sleeping for longer stretches of time and eating less often, but getting more in at each feeding.

Then one night just a few weeks later, I did her 9:00 pm and midnight feedings and put her to bed, and she stayed asleep until 7 in the morning! Of course, I freaked out, thinking something was wrong, but she was fine. Once the adrenaline wore off, I realized I'd had my first good night's sleep in weeks, and I felt amazing. I kept implementing what the book said, and she continued to sleep through the night. It was incredible.

When I went off my baby's cues, I felt like a 24/7 milk machine. That wasn't sustainable or good for either of us. She wasn't getting quality sleep, and neither was I. Getting that one full night of sleep after those first three weeks of practically no sleep was life changing. It made such a huge difference for me mentally, emotionally, and physically. I started feeling more like myself, thinking more clearly, and functioning better. As a bonus, once I was sleeping better, I started healing so much faster.

Establishing healthy sleep habits isn't just a good idea. As I found when I was learning to take care of a newborn, good sleep is absolutely essential for your fitness and wellness. In Part 3 of this book, you'll have the chance to start tracking your sleep, and I'll give you my best guidelines for creating healthy sleep habits. But first, let's talk about the impact and importance of sleep.

WHY IS SLEEP THE FIRST SHIFT?

I know you're probably wondering why I'm starting SHIFTS with sleep. Shouldn't that come last since sleep is the last thing you do in a day? No way! Sleep impacts your overall health from pretty much every angle, so it's a great foundation to start with. The sad thing is, sleep is often seen as an afterthought. It tends to be the thing people let slide the most. This is definitely true for me. Sleep is the pillar I have to work hardest to stay consistent with.

I lead a really busy life. I wake up early, and I'm going, going, going all the way up until bedtime. There's always something else to get done. Even as a kid, if I had a lot on my plate, I'd sacrifice sleep to accomplish more. What I've realized through the years is that if I don't make a consistent, conscious effort to protect my sleep as something sacred, I'll be tempted to tell myself I can sleep when I'm dead and power on…but skipping sleep is costly in the long run.

BENEFITS OF GOOD SLEEP

When you push sleep to the bottom of your priorities list, you're actually sacrificing your health. Sleep is vital to your overall quality of life. Now let's take a look at some specific areas of your body that are impacted by sleep.

Sleep and Your Brain. According to the National Institute of Neurological Disorders and Stroke, sleep plays an important role in many brain functions including your ability to learn and create new memories. When you don't get enough sleep, it can be harder to concentrate and respond to your circumstances quickly.[1] Sleep also helps regulate your metabolism and keeps you mentally sharp. But how does it do all that? Studies show that your brain uses sleep as a time to recharge and remove toxins from your system. When you don't get enough sleep, those toxins can build up and affect your mental functions.[2]

Sleep and Recovery. Sleep also helps you recover faster between training sessions. Your circadian rhythm is like your body's internal clock. It's what keeps you in sync with the natural cycle of day and night. Think of it as the rhythm your body follows to regulate sleep, wakefulness, and so much more. When your circadian rhythm is working well, you'll notice you feel energized and alert during the day and ready for restful sleep at night.

But when this rhythm is out of whack—maybe because you're staying up too late, traveling across time zones, or scrolling on your phone before bed—it can throw everything in your body off. Sleep becomes harder to get, energy levels dip, and even your metabolism and recovery can take hits. I read a study recently that talked about how even the individual cells in our skeletal muscles have circadian rhythms. When circadian rhythms are interrupted because of missed sleep, it also affects how well muscle tissue can repair and recover.[3]

Sleep, the Immune System, and Hormones. Sleep also helps keep your immune system strong and your hormones balanced. The less sleep you get, the more likely you are to get sick. In a 2015 study, researchers recorded the sleep of 164 volunteers who were exposed to the common cold. Those who had fewer than five hours of sleep in the days before being exposed were twice as likely to get sick.[4] When it comes to hormones, did you know that a lack of quality sleep can disrupt cortisol levels? That's your stress hormone, and if it's out of whack, it can lead to stubborn belly fat, fatigue, and a whole host of other issues.[5]

The good news is, you're in control of your sleep situation. You have the power to make small, manageable changes that lead to big results over time. And trust me, the results are worth it. Your body—and mind—will thank you. I recommend aiming for at least six hours a night (closer to seven or eight if possible). Keep experimenting to find what works for you.

Creating a consistent bedtime routine is one of the most overlooked yet powerful ways to support your health and well-being. I always tell my clients—it's not just about getting *more* sleep, it's about getting *better* sleep. And that starts with setting the tone before your head ever hits the pillow. If you've never had a bedtime routine, I'll give you sleep tips that will help you create one in chapter 11.

I'm a mom—I know how unpredictable things can get, so don't worry about perfection. Aim for consistency of good rest about 80–90% of the time. That's where the magic happens.

When I say sleep is foundational, I mean it. Good sleep is not only about how you feel in the morning—it's about recovery, mental clarity, and showing up as your best self in every area of your life.

Sleep isn't the only healthy practice that adds to the quality of your life. In the next section of this chapter, we're going to talk about something that's very important to our overall health—hydration.

KEY TAKEAWAYS FOR SECTION 7.1

1. **Sleep isn't optional—it's essential.** When you're rested, everything gets easier: workouts, nutrition, mindset, and recovery.
2. **Sleep is your foundation.** If you're struggling to stay consistent, don't push harder—rest smarter.
3. **Build a rhythm.** A simple, consistent sleep routine helps you think clearer, feel better, and show up stronger.

---

[1] National Institute of Neurological Disorders and Stroke (NINDS), *Brain Basics: Understanding Sleep*, accessed Feb 20, 2025, https://www.ninds.nih.gov/health-information/public-education/brain-basics/brain-basics-understanding-sleep.

[2] Andy R. Eugene and Jolanta Masiak, "The Neuroprotective Aspects of Sleep," *MEDtube Science* 3, no. 1 (2015): 35–40.

[3] *Journal of Science and Medicine in Sport*, "Volume 24, Issue 10" (October 2021): 982–987.

[4] Aric A. Prather, et al., "Behaviorally Assessed Sleep and Susceptibility to the Common Cold," *Sleep* 38, no. 9 (September 2015): 1353–1359, https://doi.org/10.5665/sleep.4968.

[5] Tae Won Kim et al., "The Impact of Sleep and Circadian Disturbance on Hormones and Metabolism," *International Journal of Endocrinology* 2015 (2015): 591729, https://doi.org/10.1155/2015/591729.

SECTION 7.2: HYDRATION

I grew up on the water from the time I was a baby. We were always out on a boat—in the ocean or on a lake—and I learned from a young age how fierce water can be and how much we must all respect its sheer force and mighty power. As I got older, I learned that water isn't just power in nature: It's power inside our bodies, too.

Did you know that the adult human body is made up of about 60% water? Water supports every major system in your body, from energy production to digestion to recovery. As we age, our water composition decreases. Staying hydrated becomes even more critical because when you're dehydrated, everything is harder—your workouts, your focus, and even your mood.

Ask me what someone could do to greatly benefit their overall fitness and wellness with the least effort and time, and I'll answer with just three words.

Drink more water.

It seems like that would be easy to do, but many people walk around like dehydrated raisins most of the time without even realizing it. Staying hydrated is absolutely necessary to our survival as humans, which is why hydration is the second pillar in my SHIFTS Framework. Your overall fitness and wellness depend on hydration, and drinking more water is one of the first daily habits I recommend for my clients to focus on when we're just getting started. As we're thinking about hydration, let's start by defining hydration.

WHAT IS HYDRATION, REALLY?

Water isn't just about quenching your thirst. In fact, in the beginning stages of dehydration, you don't even feel thirsty yet. If you wait until you're thirsty to drink water, you're most likely spending a significant part of your day dehydrated. I like to think of hydration as maintaining consistent fluid levels to keep your body in balance.

So, if hydration is keeping your body in balance, what does that look like? Well, water regulates your body temperature. Sweating helps your body stay cool. Water also helps break down food and carry nutrients to cells. Water supports your body during and after training sessions by boosting endurance, strength, and recovery. It keeps you mentally sharp, promotes supple skin and a healthy complexion, and flushes toxins out of your system.

Need a few more reasons to drink more water? Water also:

- Keeps joints lubricated
- Carries oxygen through the body
- Cushions the brain and spinal cord
- Helps maintain healthy blood pressure
- Prevents kidney damage
- Assists you in maintaining a healthy weight[1]

If it does all those good things for us, we also need to think about what occurs in our bodies when they are starved for water.

WHAT HAPPENS IF I DON'T DRINK ENOUGH WATER?

Dehydration happens when your body loses more water than

you take in and can be a potentially dangerous condition. When you're even slightly dehydrated, you're not just thirsty. Your energy depletes more easily, your recovery slows, and your immune system struggles. You can feel like your body is running uphill, working harder just to get through the day.

If we don't get enough water, our bodies will think we're being shorted and start retaining fluid as an emergency response. This leads to feeling bloated, even though you're actually dehydrated.

And if you're dehydrated long enough, your body will eventually quit functioning properly, and serious health problems can occur. Mild dehydration can cause dizziness, confusion, and exhaustion. More serious dehydration can lead to heat stroke, kidney and urinary issues, and seizures.[2] The human body can only survive for about three to five days without water. Next, let's look at what a good amount of water is as you go about your life.

HOW MUCH WATER SHOULD I DRINK DAILY?

The amount of water you need varies based on your age, weight, activity level, and climate. You should drink half your body weight in ounces of water daily at a minimum. I use a simple formula to determine how much water is needed to stay hydrated every day. The formula looks like this:

½ body weight = # of ounces of water daily

If you weigh 150 pounds, the formula looks like this:

150 / 2 = 75 ounces of water daily

Now notice that above I said that's the minimum. I personally aim for at least 96 ounces of water daily, which is almost 40 ounces more than half my body weight in ounces. I don't always hit that number, but I've noticed that when I'm consistent with this, I have more energy, fewer cravings, and even better workouts. When I'm not? My body feels sluggish, bloated, and out of sync. That's enough reason for me to up my water intake!

If you're training hard three or more days a week, it's even more critical to stay hydrated. Most active people should aim for closer to 96 to 128 ounces of water per day. People who live in hot, dry, or high elevation climates will also need more water to stay hydrated. And when you're traveling, throw an empty water bottle in your carry-on or personal item so you can fill it up once you're through TSA security. Staying hydrated boosts your immune system, making you less susceptible to illness.

Plain water is best, but if you need to shake it up from time to time, you can throw sparkling water or herb-infused water into your routine. Whatever it takes to stay hydrated. And while coffee is great and has its own health benefits, it's not a replacement for water.

I also remind my clients to listen to their bodies. If you're eating well but still feeling hungry, it might actually be thirst. Start with a glass of water instead of grabbing a snack and wait to see how you feel.

OTHER BENEFITS OF HYDRATION

Drinking water isn't just a physical act—it's an act of self-care.

Every time you reach for water, you're sending a signal that you value and want to support your body. It's empowering to know that such a simple habit can have such a profound impact on your health. When you consider that more than half of you is water, you can see why hydration is truly a cornerstone of living your strongest, healthiest, happiest life.

In Part 3 of this book, I'm going to show you how to assess and track your water intake. Then I'll give you some of my best tips for increasing your water intake over time in a way that's manageable. But before we get to that, let's talk about the other thing you put into your body—food.

KEY TAKEAWAYS FOR SECTION 7.2

1. **Hydration powers everything.** Energy, focus, digestion, mood—water supports it all. Dehydration makes everything harder and can eventually lead to severe health issues.
2. **Drink more water.** It's the fastest way to boost energy, reduce cravings, and improve recovery. Most people aren't drinking nearly enough.
3. **Don't wait to feel thirsty.** If you're thirsty, you're already dehydrated. Stay ahead by drinking consistently throughout the day.
4. **Use the simple formula.** Aim for half your body weight in ounces daily—and more if you're active or in a hot climate. Keep it simple, and make drinking water a habit.

SECTION 7.3: INTAKE AND SUSTAINABLE NUTRITION

When I was 4 or 5 years old, my dad built me a planter box to go with the mini farm in our backyard. It wasn't anything fancy—just a simple wooden frame filled with dirt—but to me, it felt like magic. Together, we planted rows of tomatoes, cucumbers, and a few other vegetables. Every day, I'd run outside to check on my little garden, watering the plants and brushing the dirt off my hands like a proud farmer.

I'll never forget the first time we harvested vegetables. I carefully picked a ripe cucumber, holding it in my tiny hands like it was a precious gem. That night, as we sliced up the cucumbers for dinner, I felt this overwhelming sense of pride. I had grown that food! I had nurtured it from a seed to something that would nourish my body. It wasn't just about the vegetables, though. It was about the process. Through that simple act of gardening, I learned patience and was rewarded with the joy of seeing my hard work turn into something real and rewarding.

I still carry those lessons with me today. Back then, I didn't realize that the empowerment I felt from growing my own food would become a cornerstone of my approach to nutrition and wellness. That little planter box wasn't just a backyard project: It was the beginning of my passion to help others take care of their bodies through sustainable nutrition.

Nutrition, much like gardening, isn't about instant results or quick fixes. It's about planting the right seeds, nurturing them with care, and having the patience to let them grow. That's what I want to share with you in this chapter—the tools and lessons that have helped me create a balanced approach to nutrition that I share every day with my clients. But before we dive into the "how," let's start with the "why."

The third pillar of my SHIFTS Framework is Intake. This refers to your nutrition—also known as what you put in your body to fuel it. My own journey with nutrition hasn't always been smooth or straightforward. In fact, it took some unexpected twists and turns, including a back injury that knocked me flat on the floor, to truly understand the power of food.

MY JOURNEY THROUGH NUTRITION

For as long as I can remember, nutrition has been important to me. In my late teens and into my twenties, I thought I had nutrition all figured out. I followed the bodybuilder-style approach, sticking to a low fat, high protein, and moderate carbs diet, all meticulously measured and planned. I was strict, disciplined, and determined to achieve peak physical fitness. On the surface, it seemed like I was doing everything "right."

But underneath, my body was telling a different story. My menstrual cycle was irregular, my energy levels fluctuated, and my face had painful acne on it. No matter how hard I trained, I couldn't seem to build muscle and take my fitness to the next level. At the time, I thought I was eating "healthy," but in reality, I wasn't giving my body the fuel it needed to thrive. That also led to my hormones being all out of whack.

Everything changed when I injured my back. I'll never forget that moment. I was doing front squats when I felt this sharp release in my lower back. I collapsed to the ground, unable to move. Lying there on the gym floor, all I could think was, *What just happened?* The pain was excruciating, and for weeks afterward, even the smallest movements were extremely uncomfortable. It was a humbling experience, to say the least.

During my recovery, I started working with a physical therapist who asked me a question that caught me completely off guard. "What does your nutrition look like?" he asked. *What do you mean?* I thought (trying not to be offended). *I eat so well! I know what I'm doing.* But the truth was, I didn't. My injury and the pain that came with it forced me to take a closer look at my diet and how it was (or wasn't) supporting my body's ability to heal.

The physical therapist suggested I try the paleo diet. At first, I dismissed it as just another fad. I had a background in nutrition, after all. I thought I knew better. But the more I read about it, the more intrigued I became. The idea of eliminating common inflammatory foods like gluten and dairy and focusing on whole, unprocessed foods made sense. Plus, I was desperate to recover and willing to try anything.

I decided to treat paleo eating as a 30-day experiment. I cut out gluten, dairy, legumes, sugar, and processed foods, focusing instead on meat, vegetables, some types of fruit, nuts, and seeds. Then I committed to blogging daily about how I felt. I took note of my sleep, mental clarity, energy levels, and mental and emotional states. I also tracked those same energy levels before, during, and after training sessions—plus I thought about how that way of eating made me feel during my training recovery.

To my surprise, the results were almost immediate. Within a week or two, I noticed a huge difference. I woke up one morning and realized I wasn't achy or sore like normal. My joints were pain free. I couldn't remember the last time I had felt that good in the morning! My energy levels were higher, my hormonal cycle regulated itself, and even my skin, something I had struggled with for years, cleared up.

By the time the 30 days were up, I was hooked. What was even better than the physical changes was that I *felt* good. For the first time in years, I was giving my body what it needed. That experiment taught me a valuable lesson. Sometimes the things we think we know about nutrition can hold us back. When we approach intake with curiosity instead of rigidity, we open ourselves up to discovering new ideas to find what truly works for us.

Since then, I've refined my approach to nutrition. I don't follow a strict paleo diet anymore, but I do use it as a foundation, and I recommend my clients prioritize whole, nutrient-dense foods and limit inflammatory foods too. I've also learned the importance of flexibility. Nutrition is about progress over perfection. It's about finding a way to fuel your body that's both effective and sustainable.

In retrospect, I realize that back injury taught me a lot, and not just about food. It taught me about resilience and humility. Plus, I learned the importance of listening to my body. I wouldn't wish that kind of injury on anyone, but in a strange way, I'm grateful for it. It opened my eyes to the power of nutrition and showed me what's possible when you truly nourish yourself from the inside out.

INTAKE = SUSTAINABLE NUTRITION

When it comes to nutrition, I've learned that sustainability is the secret sauce. It's not about following the latest trends or sticking to a diet so restrictive that it's impossible to maintain. Instead, it's about finding a way of eating that supports your goals, fits into your life, and allows you to actually enjoy your meals. Food is fuel, yes, but it's also one of the greatest joys in life. But for it to work long-term, your intake plan has to be doable long term.

For me, sustainability starts with focusing on whole, unprocessed foods. My rule of thumb is simple. If at one time it ran, swam, fell off a tree, or grew out of the ground, it's fair game. This approach, inspired by paleo, is built to emphasize foods that are nutrient-dense and as close to their natural state as possible. This approach centers around meats, vegetables, some fruits, nuts, and seeds. These foods provide your body with the vitamins, minerals, and macronutrients it needs to thrive without the inflammatory effects of processed foods, sugar, or allergens like gluten, legumes, and dairy.

Should you avoid sugar, gluten, and dairy altogether? Unless you have a food allergy, you don't have to completely cut certain foods out. Plus, you're allowed to have a treat meal now and then, and I'll talk about that further on in this chapter. If you do find your body struggles with inflammation or tends to react to certain foods, do what I did and treat your nutrition like a 30-day experiment. Start with paleo and gradually, one at a time, add in a bit of dairy or gluten back in to see how your body responds.

Even if you don't have a food allergy, food sensitivities are super common and can show up as inflammation throughout the body. If your body is highly reactive to sugar, gluten, or dairy, you may experience symptoms like:

- Nutrient malabsorption
- Bloating or water retention
- Digestive issues
- Fatigue after meals
- Brain fog, memory issues, or trouble focusing
- Headaches or migraines
- Food cravings
- Blood sugar swings or spikes
- Hormonal imbalances
- An altered gut microbiome
- Joint pain or stiffness
- Skin issues, like acne, eczema, or rashes
- Sinus congestion or running nose
- Sleep disturbances and fatigue or sluggishness
- Mood changes
- Dark circles under the eyes
- Heart rate or blood pressure changes

SHIFTING YOUR NUTRITION

When it comes to making changes to your nutrition, I always recommend starting small. Trying to overhaul everything at once is overwhelming and can make it hard to stick with your goals. That's why I encourage people to start with one simple thing, like tracking how much protein you're eating every day. By focusing on just the protein element of your nutrition first, you're building a strong base without feeling swamped by a ton of changes all at once. In Part 3 of this book, I'll give you my best tips for tracking and getting enough protein in. For now, let's talk about why protein is so important.

More Protein

Protein is the foundation of sustainable nutrition, especially if you're active. It helps with muscle repair, recovery, and stabilizing energy levels throughout the day. It even helps curb sugar cravings! The National Academy of Sports Medicine recommends 0.36 grams of protein per pound of body weight (0.8 grams of protein per kilogram of body weight).[1] I recommend aiming for more—at 1 to 1.5 grams of protein per pound of body weight. It's not always easy to get that much protein in at first, but even adding protein imperfectly makes such a huge difference. And trust me, once you start paying attention to protein, it's easier to work it into your meals.

Try to get most of your protein through actual food, like lean meats, eggs, and fish.[2] There's nothing wrong with protein shakes, and they can help fill in the gaps. But there's no substitute for the quality and satiety that whole foods provide. Start small, get consistent, and build from there.

It's all about progress, not perfection. Once you've got your protein intake dialed in, you'll be in a great spot to layer in other changes and really see the benefits of nourishing your body the right way.

More Water

Another super simple thing you can do to improve your nutrition is to drink your water. Hydration is the second pillar in my SHIFTS Framework, and I covered it in a previous section of this chapter, but it's really important in the overall context of nutrition as well. Drinking enough water helps with digestion and helps carry nutrients through your blood all over your body. Plus, hydration and protein go hand-in-hand when it comes to reducing sugar cravings.

Protein + Water = Power Duo!

Water and protein together are fundamental to the body's cellular functions and getting enough of both influences hormonal regulation, mental clarity, sleep quality, and emotional health. Talk about a power duo! Here are some additional benefits of adding more protein and water to your nutrition.

Proteins are vital to cell structure and tissue growth and form the building blocks of muscles, bones, skin, and hair.[3] Meanwhile, water helps maintain the structure and function of cells, including energy production and waste removal.[4]

Proteins act as enzymes that set off chemical reactions needed to boost metabolism and energy production,[6] while water helps regulate body temperature through perspiration and evaporation.[5]

Proteins help your body produce antibodies that protect your immune system from infections and diseases.[6] Water carries nutrients and oxygen to cells and helps remove toxins from the body.[5]

Adequate protein supports the production of hormones that regulate mood, stress responses, and cognitive functions.[7] Water aids in the transport and activation of these hormones.

Specifically, proper hydration and sufficient protein levels are associated with improved cognitive function, like better concentration and sharpened memory.[7] Dehydration and protein deficiency can impair mental clarity and focus.

Hydration affects sleep patterns, as dehydration can lead to discomfort and disrupt sleep. Proteins contribute to the production of neurotransmitters that regulate sleep cycles.

Both hydration and protein intake influence neurotransmitter function, impacting mood and emotional well-being. Imbalances can contribute to mood disorders and emotional instability. Next up, let's talk about sugar and its impact on your health.

Less Sugar

Sugar is a sneaky little troublemaker. It creates massive inflammation in your body, slows down recovery, and messes with your energy levels. Cutting back on or eliminating sugar altogether can make a world of difference, but I know that's not easy. Eating processed food makes it almost impossible to not overdo it on sugar. Don't get me started on soda and alcohol, which is often super high in added sugar. For example, the World Health Organization (WHO) recommends adults on a

2,000 calorie diet consume about 25 grams of sugar per day, yet a single can of Coke contains 44 grams.

To make matters worse, the more sugar you have in your diet, the more your body will crave it. Sugar cravings are real, especially for women. I've been known to not let anything get between me and a piece of chocolate during a certain time of the month. A four-week study on the effects of sugar on rats showed that they became quickly addicted to sugar, and their withdrawal and relapse symptoms were similar to what a person who is addicted to drugs experiences.[8]

Here's the good news though. When you focus on hitting your protein goals and drinking enough water, sugar cravings tend to fade. Protein helps balance your blood sugar and keeps you satisfied, so you're not constantly reaching for something sweet. And when you do want a treat, there are plenty of healthier options, like berries, sweet potatoes, or clementines, which are lower on the glycemic index and still satisfy that sweet tooth.

Something really cool happens when sugar or complex carbohydrates are paired with protein though—something that's a game-changer when it comes to fueling your body, improving your recovery, and optimizing your performance. Sugar helps drive protein absorption by spiking insulin, which moves amino acids straight to your muscles for faster repair and growth.[9] If you're training hard and need to replenish glycogen stores (think of glycogen as your body's fuel reserve tank for quick energy storage), combining carbs with protein post-workout speeds up recovery and reduces muscle breakdown.[10] But the benefits don't stop there.

When sugar is eaten alongside protein, the presence of protein helps stabilize the blood sugar response by slowing digestion. Slower digestion minimizes the potential blood sugar spike that would come from eating simple sugars on their own and leads to a more balanced insulin response.[11] Inside your body, sugar attaches to proteins to form glycoproteins, which help proteins travel where they need to go, fold into the right shape, and be absorbed better for use inside your body.[12]

When sugar is consumed without being paired with protein, however, it can have various not-so-great effects on the body.[13] Your blood sugar spikes, which can lead to a crash or drop in blood sugar levels later, often leaving you feeling tired, irritable, and hungry again. When your blood sugar spikes, it triggers your pancreas to produce more insulin. High insulin levels can encourage fat storage, particularly in the abdominal area.[14] Over time, consistent blood sugar spikes can lead to an increased risk for type 2 diabetes. Blood sugar spikes can also cause your body to release cortisol, a stress hormone. High cortisol can have a negative impact on your mood, sleep, and stress levels.

Need more evidence that sugar without protein is a troublemaker? Sugar without protein can increase systemic inflammation that increases your risk for cardiovascular disease, joint issues, and even mental health disorders like depression.[15] Without protein, the body may not feel full or satisfied after a sugary meal or snack, leading to overeating. High sugar intake without the balancing effects of protein and fiber can negatively affect the gut microbiome and lead to digestive issues and bloating.[16]

Bottom line? This isn't about "good" or "bad" foods. It's about paying attention to what fuels your body smarter. Whether you're looking to maximize muscle growth, recover faster, or just get more from your nutrition, pairing protein with the right carbohydrates can take your performance to the next level.[19]

Want a downloadable nutrition resource you can access from anywhere? Turn to the Resources section of this book for instructions on how to access my Phase 1 Nutrition Guide as well as my Phase 1 Nutrition "In a Nutshell," a short, printable guide to intake that you can hang on your fridge.

What About Supplements?

In a perfect world, everyone would be able to get all their nutrients, vitamins, and minerals from food. That's the goal anyway. But, it's not always possible. Thankfully, supplements are a great way to enhance your nutrition and fill in any gaps. For supplements, I recommend that everyone take creatine, a probiotic, and a multi-vitamin. It's also helpful to visit your health professional and have your blood panels done to see if you have any vitamin or mineral deficiencies. Your doctor can then recommend the right foods and supplements for you.

While supplements can help support your body on a cellular level, your mindset around food is just as important, even when you're thinking about having a treat.

EMBRACE TREAT (NOT CHEAT) MEALS

Sustainable nutrition isn't just about *what* you eat. It's also about how you approach eating. I've never been a fan of labeling foods as "good" or "bad," and I don't like the term "cheat meal." That mindset feels restrictive and full of guilt, and that's the last thing you need when you're working toward sustainable nutrition goals.

Instead, I encourage you to incorporate "treat meals" into your life. A treat meal isn't about throwing your goals out the window. It's about enjoying something you love in a controlled, intentional way that doesn't sideline your overall nutrition. For me, treat meals often fall on rest or active recovery days, and I plan them in advance.

For example, if you've been consistent all week, schedule a treat meal and plan out what you'll have. Maybe it's pasta, a burger, or a slice of cake. Planning for a treat meal will help you enjoy it guilt-free, and this is a fun way to reward yourself for your hard work. Just remember, it's a treat meal, not a treat *day*.

The beauty of this approach is that it allows for flexibility. There will be birthdays, holidays, and moments when you just want to eat pizza or enjoy a glass of wine. You don't want to take all the fun out of your life when it comes to food. Sustainable nutrition is about making choices that align with your goals *most of the time* while still leaving room in your life for the joy and connection that food brings. If you aim for consistency in your intake 80% of the time, you're doing great!

Remember, SHIFTS is all about creating healthy habits that last a lifetime. Sustainable nutrition will nourish you in a way that's simple, consistent, and empowering—not force you into such a state of restriction that it's impossible to stick to your plan. When you break your approach to food down into simple, actionable steps, like starting by increasing protein and building from there, nutrition doesn't have to feel overwhelming.

KEY TAKEAWAYS FOR SECTION 7.3

1. **Nutrition is a long game.** It's not about diets. It's about building a lasting, supportive relationship with food.
2. **Stick to real food.** If it ran, swam, flew, grew out of the ground, or fell off a tree, it's a good choice. Keep food choices simple and close to nature.
3. **Meal prep matters.** Batch cook basics like protein, veggies, and carbs once a week. It saves time, money, and stress.
4. **Balance your plate.** Aim for protein and complex carbs at every meal. Eating four to five times a day (or every three hours or so) keeps energy steady and cravings low.
5. **Prioritize protein.** It supports fullness, muscle, and recovery. Focus on whole foods, and supplement protein in things like shakes only when needed.
6. **Enjoy treat meals.** Planned indulgences help you stay consistent—no guilt required.

[1] Fabio Carr. "The Power of Protein: How Much, What Kind, and When." *NASM Blog*, May 27, 2022. https://blog.nasm.org/nutrition/power-protein.

[2] Harvard T.H. Chan School of Public Health. "Protein." *The Nutrition Source*. Accessed August 11, 2025. https://nutritionsource.hsph.harvard.edu/what-should-you-eat/protein.

[3] Janice R. Hermann. *Protein and the Body*. Stillwater: Oklahoma State University Extension. Accessed August 11, 2025. https://extension.okstate.edu/fact-sheets/print-publications/t/protein-and-the-body-t-3163.pdf.https://extension.okstate.edu/fact-sheets/print-publications/t/protein-and-the-body-t-3163.pdf.

[4] Jessica Migala, Abbott Nutrition, *What Is Hydration on a Cellular Level and Why Is It Important?* n.d. https://www.nutritionnews.abbott/healthy-living/diet-wellness/What-Is-Hydration-on-a-Cellular-Level-and-Why-Is-It-Important

[5] Mayo Clinic Health System, *Water: Essential to Your Body (Video)*, N.d., https://www.mayoclinichealthsystem.org/hometown-health/speaking-of-health/water-essential-to-your-body-video

[6] Jillian Kubala, 2021, "What Are the Functions of Protein?" *Healthline*, June 16, 2021. https://www.healthline.com/nutrition/functions-of-protein.

[7] David Benton and Hayley Donohoe, 2011, "The Influence of Protein Intake on Mental Performance," *Nutrition Research Reviews* 24 (1): 169–82. https://doi.org/10.1017/S0954422411000086.

[8] CH Wideman, GR Nadzam, and HM Murphy, 2005, "Implications of an animal model of sugar addiction, withdrawal and relapse for human health", *Nutritional Neuroscience*, 8(5–6), 269–276. https://doi.org/10.1080/10284150500485221

[9] Satoshi Fujita, Blake B. Rasmussen, Jerson G. Cadenas, James J. Grady, and Elena Volpi, 2006, "Effect of Insulin on Human Skeletal Muscle Protein Synthesis Is Modulated by Insulin-Induced Changes in Muscle Blood Flow and Amino Acid Availability," *American Journal of Physiology – Endocrinology and Metabolism* 291 (4): E624–31. https://doi.org/10.1152/ajpendo.00271.2005.

[10] Chris Poole, Colin Wilborn, Lem Taylor, and Chad Kerksick, 2010, "The Role of Post-Exercise Nutrient Administration on Muscle Protein Synthesis and Glycogen Synthesis," *Journal of Sports Science & Medicine* 9 (3): 354–63. https://doi.org/10.51797/jssm.354361.

[11] Jing Ma, Julie E. Stevens, Kimberly Cukier, Anne F. Maddox, Judith M. Wishart, Peter M. Clifton, Michael Horowitz, and Christopher K. Rayner, 2009, "Effects of a Protein Preload on Gastric Emptying, Glycemia, and Gut Hormones After a Carbohydrate Meal in Diet-Controlled Type 2 Diabetes," *Diabetes Care* 32, no. 9: 1600–02. https://doi.org/10.2337/dc09-0723.

[12] Stefan W. Stoll, Jessica L. Johnson, Ajay Bhasin, Andrew Johnston, Johann E.

Gudjonsson, Laure Rittié, and James T. Elder, 2010, "Metalloproteinase-Mediated, Context-Dependent Function of Amphiregulin and HB-EGF in Human Keratinocytes and Skin." *Journal of Investigative Dermatology* 130 (1): 295–304. https://doi.org/10.1038/jid.2009.211.

[13] Kris Gunnars, BSc. *Healthline*, 2021, February 17, "12 Tips to Prevent Blood Sugar Spikes", https://www.healthline.com/nutrition/blood-sugar-spikes

[14] TM Wolever, JB Miller, 1995), "Sugars and blood glucose control." Am J Clin Nutr. 1995 Jul;62(1 Suppl):212S-221S; discussion 221S-227S. doi: 10.1093/ajcn/62.1.212S. PMID: 7598079.

[15] Howard E. LeWine, M.D. Harvard Health Publishing. 2020. "The Sweet Danger of Sugar." Retrieved from https://www.health.harvard.edu/heart-health/the-sweet-danger-of-sugar

[16] Kerri M Gillespie, Eva Kemps, Melanie J White, Selena E Bartlett. 2023. "The Impact of Free Sugar on Human Health—A Narrative Review", *Nutrients*: 15(4):889. doi: 10.3390/nu15040889. PMID: 36839247; PMCID: PMC9966020.

[17] B. D. Roy, M. A. Tarnopolsky, J. D. MacDougall, J. Fowles, and K. E. Yarasheski, 1997, "Effect of Glucose Supplement Timing on Protein Metabolism after Resistance Training." *Journal of Applied Physiology* 82 (6): 1882–88. https://doi.org/10.1152/jappl.1997.82.6.1882.

SECTION 7.4: FITNESS

I've worked with many clients over the years, and each one has helped me grow as a coach and as a person. Like I shared earlier, one client I'll never forget came to me after suffering a stroke that left him with limited use of the entire left side of his body. It was unlike anything I'd ever encountered as a coach. I'd worked with athletes who were amputees or wheelchair users, but this was different. With those athletes, we could still rely on the functionality of their other limbs. But with this client, everything was unilateral—we had to build strength and mobility on one side while working creatively to engage the other.

We started small, exploring ways he could perform basic movements like push-ups, squats, and even modified pull-ups. It took serious out-of-the-box thinking where we had to adjust for form and build up from the most foundational movements. Every rep he completed was a triumph, not just because of the physical effort, but because it signified progress and proof that his body was capable of adapting and growing stronger. Over time, he began performing exercises like ring dips and barbell movements that had at first felt like impossible goals. Watching him regain his strength and confidence reminded me of the resilience and adaptability of the human body, mind, and spirit.

I've also had the privilege of working alongside a coach who trained a blind adaptive athlete determined to master CrossFit. Seeing this client tackle movements like wall balls and double-unders was beyond inspiring. The challenge wasn't just physical—it was logistical, too. Without sight, she had to rely entirely on tactile and verbal cues to understand form, rhythm, and spatial awareness. It wasn't easy, but her determination and willingness to trust her coaches and her body were incredible.

These experiences taught me that fitness is for everyone, no matter where you're starting from. The human body and spirit are capable of extraordinary things when given the opportunity. It's not about fitting into a mold or following a one-size-fits-all program. It's about finding what works for you, embracing your unique challenges, and proving to yourself that you can do hard things. Fitness—the fourth pillar of my SHIFTS Framework—isn't just about physical strength. It's about reclaiming confidence and the freedom to move all while building habits that support you not just today, but for the rest of your life.

Let's start with the point you're at right now. Once we set the foundation, one step at a time, you will be able to build strength for life.

MEETING YOURSELF WHERE YOU ARE

One of the most important lessons I've learned as a coach, and in my own fitness journey, is that the best place to start is always right where you are. Don't try to start where you think you *should* be or where someone else is. The truth is, there's no "perfect" place to begin. What matters is that you decide to take action and give yourself permission to grow at your own pace.

So where should you start? When I work with clients, one of the first things I do is get a sense of who they are not just physically, but mentally and emotionally. Fitness isn't a one-size-fits-all journey. Your approach depends on so many factors, like your goals, your personality, your current conditioning, any physical limitations, and even the demands of your daily life. Are you someone who likes to go all in and push yourself to extremes, only to burn out after a few weeks? Or are you hesitant, unsure if you're ready to commit fully? Wherever you fall on that spectrum, the key is to find a structure that actually *supports you* and that is doable long term—without you feeling overwhelmed.

For fitness beginners, I always recommend starting gradually, one step at a time. Maybe it's committing to one or two structured workouts each week, combined with light, consistent movement on your own two to three times each week. Take a 30-minute walk, hit a yoga session, or go on a bike ride. For the first two or three weeks, focus on one simple thing—creating the habit of showing up. You don't need to do anything extreme or complicated. Just focus on moving your body in ways that feel good and are sustainable.

For example, one client I worked with hadn't done any structured exercise in years. We started with just two days of training together, focusing on foundational bodyweight movements like squats, push-ups, and planks. On the other days, I encouraged her to take walks in her neighborhood or ride her bike with her kids. No fancy equipment, no intense regimens. Within a few weeks, she felt more confident, her energy had improved, and she started looking forward to her workouts. Next, we began layering in more sessions when she was ready. That's the power of starting where you are and building from there.

It's not just about your physical conditioning, though. Fitness is as much about mindset as it is about movement. We'll talk more about the particulars of that in the next section of this chapter. For now, keep in mind that if your schedule is packed or you're dealing with stress, it's important to acknowledge that and set realistic expectations for yourself. Trying to do too much too soon can lead to frustration and burnout, and that's the opposite of what we want. Fitness should feel like an investment in yourself, not another item on your to-do list that drains your energy.

And here's another important thing to keep in mind. Your starting point isn't a reflection of your worth or your potential. It's simply a snapshot of where you are today. Maybe you're coming back to fitness after having kids, or maybe you're starting for the first time in your life. Wherever you're starting, the most important thing is to meet yourself with kindness and grace. Sustainable progress is about showing up consistently and taking small, steady steps forward.

If you're not sure where to begin, pick a physical activity you enjoy or something you're curious about. Love being outside? Go for walks or hikes. Like structure? Try a group fitness class or work with a trainer. The goal isn't to find the "perfect" workout. The goal is to find something that challenges you so that you can stick with it and build on over time.

Remember, your fitness journey is unique to you. It's not about comparing yourself to anyone else or trying to match someone else's pace. No matter where you're starting, you're taking the first step toward a stronger, healthier, happier version of yourself, and that's something to be proud of.

SETTING A GOAL AND CORRESPONDING TRAINING FOCUSES

Speaking of taking steps, let's talk about where to begin. If it's been a while or you're new to physical fitness, here's what I recommend to get you off to a solid start: set an overall goal, then break that goal down into training focuses for each session. This is something I do with every client when we start working together, then again at regular intervals as they achieve a goal and set new ones.

Having both long-term and short-term goals is important. Your long-term goals will help you stay aligned with your "why," which is the deeper core reason behind pursuing and maintaining a fit lifestyle. Fun, short-term goals keep us on the path while enjoying our fitness and ability to be active, and testing ourselves in different ways using the fitness we have built through consistent training.

Goals and training focus work together. If you think of a goal as the destination or result you're aiming for, then your training focus for each workout is a step on the roadmap that gets you closer. Both are crucial, and understanding how they work together can completely change the way you approach your fitness journey.

Goals are the big-picture benchmarks that give you direction and motivation. Maybe your goal is to run a 5K, to build muscle, or simply to feel stronger and more confident in your body for the rest of your life. Goals help you see where you're headed and keep you moving forward, even on the tough days.

Goals aren't enough on their own, however. Take the goal of running a 5K, for example. This is a great goal, but how will you go from who you are today to someone who can run a 5K? Without a clear, personalized plan to follow, you'll feel stuck or frustrated. But add in a training focus for each step of your journey toward running a 5K and things will become clearer.

Training focus is about having a specific intention for each workout or training session. When I create individually designed programs for my clients, each training session has an intention and a focus for the day that is a building block in their overall program.

Instead of just showing up and going through the motions, a training focus helps you stay mindful of what you're doing and why you're doing it. When you train with focus, every session becomes a building block that moves you closer to your goal. Your training focus for the goal of running a 5K might include things like building endurance by maintaining a steady pace during a long run, working on speed intervals to improve your time, or strengthening your core and legs to support your running mechanics.

Let's look at another example of goal versus training focus, this time using the goal of improving your body composition or your body's makeup of fat, bone, water, and muscle. This is a great goal because the more muscle you have, the faster or higher your metabolism will naturally stay even while at rest. More muscle = increased fat loss! Your training focus for this goal might be increasing the load on your squats or deadlifts to build strength and lean mass, dialing in your form and technique on key movements, or incorporating higher-intensity sessions to boost your metabolism.

The beauty of having a training focus for each session is that it helps keep things flexible and manageable. Although your goal stays consistent, you can change your training focus based on your health, energy levels, and what your body needs. Some days, your focus might be on moving with perfect form and control. Other days, it might be about pushing your limits with heavier weights or a faster pace. The key is to approach each session with intention, rather than just checking a workout off your list.

How Goals and Training Focus Work Together

Your goal is the "why," and your training focus is the "how." Together, they create a system that keeps you motivated and on track. Without a goal, your workouts can feel aimless, like you're working hard for no reason. And without a training focus, your goal can start to feel out of reach because you don't have a plan to break it down into manageable steps.

One of the most common mistakes I see people make is focusing only on the end result. They get so caught up in the goal—whether it's hitting a specific weight, finishing a race, or reaching a performance milestone—that they forget to find joy in the process. But the truth is, progress happens in the details. It's in the way you approach each workout, each rep, and each choice you make along the way.

Remember, fitness and wellness are about quality of life and becoming the best version of yourself. Keep your "why" in mind for long-term consistency and longevity. Goals are great, but don't lose sight of your overall why. Your "why" must be even deeper than a single stand-alone goal like running a 5K or doing a weightlifting competition.

How to Set a Training Focus

If you're working with a coach, they'll usually guide you through this process. They'll design your programming with specific goals in mind and outline the training focus for each session. For example, your coach might tell you, "Today's focus is on maintaining tempo in your squats" or "Your goal is to build volume while maintaining proper form."

Over time, as you gain experience and awareness, you'll be able to set your own training focus, even within a structured program. Setting a training focus or intention is super specific to the actual program design for each piece in each training session. The focus can vary greatly from day to day or training session to training session, depending on your goals. Here are some examples of things you could use as training focuses:

Improved form and technique: Focus on moving with precision and control in the best form possible, even if that means less weight or fewer reps.

Better pacing: Find a challenging pace throughout your first set and aim to match or even beat yourself by even one second each following set. Setting a goal for the pace you want to hold on each set and focusing on that rather than how your body feels can help you push through the temporary discomfort.

An example of improving your pacing might look like part of one of my recent training sessions. Every four minutes I set a goal to do:

- 12 toes to bar
- 16 burpee box jump-overs
- 12 toes to bar

My goal was to do four sets with a target time from 2:15 to 2:45 with a time cap at 3 minutes with a 1-minute rest between sets.

The goal was to move at a challenging pace while also aiming to keep it as consistent as possible across all four sets. With toes to bar, it is tough. It is common to hit a wall, as it requires quite a bit of muscle endurance to maintain the pace you started with on that first round while factoring in the amount of volume and the intensity level of both movements. You must be able to hit each set within the target time—or at least under the time cap—to ensure the allotted rest and recovery time between sets while achieving and maintaining the intended intensity and power output. The forced 1-minute rest is to allow for "some" recovery between sets while still making the training challenging. Pushing hard through repeated efforts without full recovery, while volume and fatigue build over time, keeps you focused and reinforces the goal of the workout.

My sets were 2:06, 2:16, 2:33, 2:42. Even though my times got slower each set, I was happy to hit within the target time each set. I was also happy with my ability to move as quickly as I could while holding a consistent, quick pace on my burpee box jump-overs, even when I hit a wall on my toes to bar around the end of my third set, as it was my first workout back after being sick the past few days so I gave myself grace.

Increased strength: Gradually build your load when lifting while maintaining proper technique and movement mechanics.

Skill development: Practice various progressions for movements like pull-ups or handstands, with a strong emphasis on the little details within training proper body position, shapes, technique, etc.

Active recovery: Move with intention and light effort to support recovery through blood flow, low to no eccentric loading (focusing on cyclical movement patterns such as swimming, rowing, and biking), mobility, and flexibility. Eccentric loading offers low to no impact on your body and joints.

The key is to approach each session with a clear purpose. Even on days when you're feeling tired or unmotivated, having a focus helps you stay engaged and get something meaningful out of your workout. If you're new to setting a training focus, don't overthink it. Start with one small intention for each session. Maybe it's something as simple as "maintain great form" or "focus on breathing." Over time, you'll get better at identifying what your body needs and how to structure your workouts to support your goals while addressing those needs.

BODYWEIGHT BASICS

When it comes to fitness, I'm a big believer in starting with the basic bodyweight movements—what I call functional gymnastics—because they are the most effective way to build the strong foundation and body awareness needed for all other types of movement, no matter your starting point. And the best part? Bodyweight movements are accessible to everyone. You don't need a gym membership, expensive equipment, or a lot of time. You can do them at home, on the beach, in a park, or wherever you have space. All you need is your body, a little bit of consistency, and a willingness to learn. Whether you're just getting started with fitness, looking to reset and strengthen your fundamentals, or wanting to train for a specific event or challenge, mastering these movements sets the stage for everything else.

One of the biggest mistakes I see people make is trying to skip the basics. They want to dive straight into lifting heavy weights or doing complex workouts without mastering the fundamentals first. But trust me—putting in the time to build a solid foundation of strength and flexibility will pay off in the long run. You'll move better, recover faster, and be able to take on more advanced challenges with confidence. You'll also have a more resilient body, possess far greater body awareness, and be less prone to injury.

When you start with these movements, you're creating a foundation that supports everything else in your fitness journey. These exercises teach you proper technique and form, basic movement mechanics, and how to move well, build strength, and improve your stability and mobility. And because they're scalable, you can adjust them to match your current fitness level and progress as you get stronger. The underlying theme and tone of bodyweight training is to build a rocksolid, bulletproof core. We are, and will only stay, as strong and healthy as our core (which we also refer to in the fitness world as midline or trunk).

Bodyweight training isn't just about building strength. It's about strength, balance, coordination, agility, flexibility, and accuracy. That's more than half of the ten general physical skills CrossFit focuses on. You could even argue that bodyweight training hits the rest of these skills—cardio/respiratory endurance, stamina, power, speed—too.

If you can't move your own body efficiently and effectively, adding external weights or complexity isn't going to help. It'll actually increase your risk of injury. That's why I always start clients with bodyweight movements, focusing on mastering the essentials with proper form and technique before we layer in more advanced work.

Bodyweight exercises teach you how to connect with your body. They help you build strength, stability, and coordination in ways that carry over into everyday life. Think about it—every time you sit down, stand up, reach for something, pick something up, or climb a set of stairs, you're essentially doing a version of an upper body push or pull or a lower body push or pull. By training these movements with intention and proper technique, you're not just getting stronger, you're improving how you move through life.

In the fitness section of chapter 11, you'll find detailed descriptions of several of my top movements for effectively building a solid strength base and movement foundation.

These descriptions will help you execute the movements and foundational body positions and shapes with proper form and technique. I also include my movement standards and benchmarks for knowing when you're ready to progress beyond the basic movement and how to uplevel the movements for greater results. You'll also have the chance to grab a free 7-day training plan, complete with a downloadable guide and videos for each movement when you access the Resources section of this book.

HOW TO KNOW WHEN YOU'RE READY FOR MORE

One of the most exciting parts of any fitness journey is hitting that point where you feel ready to take things to the next level. Progression is a natural and essential part of growth, but you don't want to force it, especially since you're in this for the long term. To stay healthy while progressing, it's super important to remember to focus on building upon the foundation you've created in a way that's sustainable and aligned with your goals.

Progression starts with developing consistency. Start by showing up and being active regularly, building healthy habits, and creating a solid base to grow from. If you've been sticking to your routine, recovering well, and feeling stronger, that's a great sign you're ready to explore the next step. Here are some of the key indicators I look for when helping clients determine if it's time to level up their training:

You're recovering well between sessions. If you're no longer feeling sore for days after your workouts and you're bouncing back quickly, it's a good sign your body is adapting. You're ready to safely handle more intensity, volume, or frequency—and a heavier load. If soreness is still a constant, it might mean you need to focus on more hydration, more protein, and more sleep before increasing your load.

Your workouts feel manageable. When you're completing your sessions with good energy and form, and they no longer feel as challenging as they used to, that's your body telling you it's ready for more. This could mean increasing your intensity level, the load you're lifting, adding a few more reps, or taking on a slightly longer session.

You've mastered the basics. Progression isn't just about doing more. It's also about doing what you've been doing well. If you've nailed the fundamentals, like squats, push-ups, and planks, and you're moving with confidence and control, it might be time to add a layer. This could include adding a barbell or some sort of external load or a resistance band or progressing to more advanced movements, like a jump squat or side plank.

You're feeling stronger and more confident. Progression is as much about mindset as it is about physical readiness. If you're feeling excited about your workouts and confident in your abilities, it's a great time to challenge yourself with something new. On the flip side, if you're feeling unsure or overwhelmed, it's okay to stay where you are and build more consistency before moving forward.

You're asking for more. One of the clearest signs you're ready is when you find yourself wanting to do more. Maybe you're thinking, *What else can I do on my off days?* or *Could I add in another training session?* If you're eager to push yourself, that's a great sign you've built a solid foundation and are ready to progress.

WAYS TO PROGRESS

Once you've recognized that you're ready for more, there are several ways to take things up a notch. Choose from the list below, but make sure you only add one of these at a time:

Increase training frequency. If you're currently working out two to three days a week, try adding another session. This could be a structured strength day, a high-intensity interval workout, or even an active recovery session like yoga or swimming. The key is to add gradually. Don't jump from two days to five overnight. Give your body, life rhythm, and mind time to adjust.

Add intensity. Intensity doesn't always mean going harder or faster. It could mean lifting heavier weights, working on tempo (slowing down or speeding up), or incorporating interval training to challenge your cardiovascular system.

Introduce variety. Progression isn't just about doing more of the same thing. It's also about exploring new movements, formats, or trying new sports. If you've been focusing on bodyweight movements, consider adding free weights or resistance bands. Variety keeps your workouts challenging and fun.

Focus on skill development. For example, you might work on improving your pull-up technique, mastering handstands, or perfecting your squat depth. Skill-based goals keep you motivated and give you a sense of accomplishment.

Set new goals. Progress often comes with a shift in goals. Once you've achieved one goal, take some time to reflect on what's next. Maybe you feel comfortable having trained for a 5K and want to work toward a 10K. Maybe there's a fitness competition you have your eye on. Setting new goals helps you stay motivated and gives your training a clear direction.

HOW TO KNOW IF YOU'RE PUSHING TOO HARD

While progress is exciting, it's important to listen to your body and know when to pull back. Feeling sore when starting a new program or changing up your training in some capacity is normal, and it is okay to still workout. This is especially true in the first one to three weeks. After the initial four to six weeks, if you're feeling a tender-to-the-touch type of soreness or an intense soreness that is lasting for more than one to two days post-training session on a regular basis, then something is up and needs to be addressed.

If you're constantly sore, feeling fatigued, or struggling to recover between sessions, it might be a sign that you're doing too much too soon—and a warning that you need to check the rest of your SHIFTS pillars. Rest and recovery are just as important as training, and sometimes scaling back is exactly what your body needs to keep making progress.

If you're unsure whether you're ready to progress, take a step back and evaluate your overall recovery. Are you staying hydrated? Eating enough protein? Getting quality sleep? The other SHIFT pillars can play a huge role in how your body adapts to training, and they're often the missing pieces when progression stalls.

STRENGTH FOR LIFE

When I think about fitness, I don't just think about how much weight you can lift, how fast you can run, or how many reps you can do. Those things are great benchmarks, and I love seeing clients hit their goals. But what really excites me, and what really matters to my clients, is what fitness gives you beyond the gym. It gives you the ability to stay active, flexible, mobile, and strong in the future.

Strength for life is about being able to move through your days with confidence and ease. It's the ability to carry your groceries up the stairs, pick up your kids or grandkids without strain, or take on a new adventure without hesitation. It's about longevity, staying active and capable as you age, and giving yourself the tools to stay independent and resilient for as long as possible. The muscle and movement you build today will support you for decades to come. Staying fit is the best way to encourage longevity. Strength and fitness protect you against illness, injury, and the wear and tear of life.

And let's not forget the joy that comes with fitness. There's something magical about feeling strong in your body—about surprising yourself with what you can do—and about setting a goal and crushing it. Experiencing physical strength is empowering, it's uplifting, and it carries over into every area of your life. When you're stronger physically, you feel stronger mentally. When you feel capable in your workouts, you feel capable in your career, your relationships, and your day-to-day life.

KEY TAKEAWAYS FOR SECTION 7.4

1. **Fitness is for every body.** No matter your ability, age, or starting point, your body can adapt and grow stronger.
2. **Modify the movement, not the goal.** Adjust exercises to fit your needs. There's always a way to keep moving forward.
3. **Train for life.** Strength isn't just about numbers. Being strong means you can do what you love with confidence and ease for *longer.*
4. **Start small.** One step taken and maintained consistently leads to progress and discipline. Confidence is built through progress, discipline, and consistency.
5. **Use what you've got.** No gym? No problem. Move in ways that work for you. Keep it fun, keep it simple, and stay steady.

SECTION 7.5: THOUGHTS AND MINDSET

If I've learned anything from my journey with fitness and wellness, it's that everything begins with mindset.

Back in 2009, when I stepped into a CrossFit gym for the first time, I had no idea what I was walking into. I'd spent years training as a gymnast, lifting weights, and bodybuilding, so I figured I was strong, agile, and ready for just about anything. But let me tell you, I was not prepared for how humbling and empowering that first workout would be. Within minutes of starting, I realized I was in for a bigger challenge than I anticipated. My lungs were burning, my muscles were screaming, and my brain kept telling me, *This is way harder than it looks.*

And yet, I kept going.

Something happened during that workout. It wasn't just about pushing through the physical discomfort or finishing the workout. It was about realizing I was stronger than I thought, and not just physically, but mentally too. Because of CrossFit, I learned that even when my body feels like giving up, I can keep moving because my mindset is strong.

That realization was *life changing.*

CrossFit taught me how to embrace being uncomfortable and to push through limits I didn't even know I had while finding joy in the process of getting stronger. And that's something I carry with me to this day in my own training and in the way I coach others. What surprised me the most, though, was how much my mental resilience grew alongside my physical strength. Showing up for those workouts day after day, choosing to voluntarily face challenges, and pushing myself to new levels wasn't just about fitness. It was about building confidence, grit, and a belief in my ability to handle whatever life throws my way.

HOW TO BE READY FOR ANYTHING

Another benefit of training your mindset daily is you'll be ready for anything. I love this mentality. It's why I'm drawn to CrossFit and functional fitness. And it's not just about physical fitness. It's about mental fitness, too. This is something I learned from my first CrossFit coach. I started going to a gym when I still lived in my home state of Texas back in August of 2009. It was owned by a strong, amazing lady in her late 40s or early 50s. She was super fit and consistent—and she pushed us. In fact, no style of training I had ever done up to that point had pushed me as far mentally as her workouts did.

Every day is different in CrossFit. The movements and intensity levels are constantly varied from day to day and are always guaranteed to be super fun, and maybe a little soul crushing if you're into that sort of thing.

Yet, as hard as it was, it was so good. For the first time, I realized the connection between pushing myself physically and growing mentally. I realized how much of an impact my internal self-talk created during the workouts that I wasn't sure I could finish. I remember one specific workout where I was super fatigued and extremely uncomfortable. My internal self-talk started.

I don't know if I can finish this workout. Why am I doing this to myself?

The moment that thought crossed my mind, I remembered why I was doing CrossFit, and my mindset changed. I started to focus only on the next rep, then the next. And inside my head, I became my own cheerleader.

You're doing great! You can do this. You are so strong.

I finished that workout—and the next one—and the next. I improved and got consistently better week after week. In fact, within the first three weeks, I started seeing results like I had never seen in my body before. But the results that couldn't be physically seen—those were even greater. I sent that woman an email to tell her how grateful I was for her coaching. I wanted her to know that I felt so much stronger, physically and mentally. Her work as my coach changed my life.

YOUR INNER COACH...OR YOUR INNER CRITIC?

The way you talk to yourself matters. Your internal dialogue, or the constant stream of thoughts running through your mind, can either be your greatest ally or your biggest obstacle. The good news is, you have the power to choose which one it will be.

When I started CrossFit, I had no idea how much my mental conversations would come into play. I was caught off guard by how much I had to battle my own thoughts. But then, something shifted. I realized I didn't have to listen to the voice telling me to give up. I could choose to replace those thoughts with a different voice that encouraged me, pushed me, and reminded me why I started in the first place. Instead of focusing on how much further I had to go or how hard it felt in that moment, I started mentally telling myself, *Just one more rep. Just keep moving. You can do this.*

You know what? It worked. Every time I chose to override the unhelpful self-talk with something positive, I found strength I didn't even know I had.

Self-talk is incredibly powerful because it shapes how you approach challenges. It's the difference between mentally checking out or quitting when things get tough and pushing through to see what you're capable of. When you let your inner critic take the wheel, it magnifies your doubts and fears, making every obstacle feel insurmountable. But when you lean into your inner coach, you create a mindset of resilience and possibility. You start to see challenges as opportunities to grow rather than reasons to give up.

Pay attention to the things you're saying to yourself, especially in difficult moments. Are you encouraging yourself, or are you tearing yourself down? If you notice that your inner dialogue is unpleasant, don't get discouraged. We've all been there. Acknowledge that your words aren't helping you and remind yourself that you have the power to change how you are speaking to yourself. Here are some tips that have helped me:

Focus only on the next step. When you're in the middle of a tough workout or other challenging situation, it's easy to get overwhelmed by the big picture. Instead of thinking about how far you have to go, focus on the next step or the next rep. Think to yourself, *One rep at a time.* Breaking tasks down into smaller pieces makes them feel more manageable and keeps you moving forward.

Reframe the discomfort. Discomfort isn't your enemy. It's a sign that you're growing. A friend of mine once sat next to author and speaker Jocko Willink at a dinner. She asked him how he overcame negative thoughts that popped up during training as a Navy Seal. His response surprised her. He said he doesn't have negative thoughts, and then explained that there are no positive or negative thoughts. They're just thoughts, and you have the power to control them. When you start to feel uncomfortable, instead of thinking, "This hurts; I can't do it," try reframing it as, "This is hard, but I'm getting stronger. This is where the magic happens." You can also try not thinking any thoughts at all. Finding stillness of mind in the middle of tough moments isn't easy, but I've found that meditation helps with this. It calms the mind and saves energy in tough workouts. I've also learned that the moments when you want to quit are the moments when you have the most to gain by seeing it through, whatever you're doing .

Use encouraging mantras. I've developed a few go-to phrases that I repeat to myself when I need a mental boost. Things like, "I've got this," or "one more rep," or "strong and steady." These mantras might sound cheesy or simple, but they're incredibly effective at keeping me focused and grounded before my mind starts to have other ideas.

Talk to yourself like a friend. Imagine if a close friend came to you and said they were struggling. Would you tell them to quit? Would you point out all the reasons they can't succeed? Of course not! You'd encourage them, remind them of their strength, and cheer them on. So why not extend that same kindness to yourself? When you catch yourself being overly critical, ask, "What would I say to a friend in this situation?" Then, say that to yourself.

The beauty of self-talk is that it's a skill you can practice and strengthen, just like any muscle. Every time you choose to reframe thoughts or use encouraging words instead of tearing yourself down, you're building that mental muscle. Over time, it becomes second nature. You'll start to approach challenges with more confidence, knowing that you can handle whatever comes your way.

Every time you push through a moment of doubt, you're proving to yourself that you're stronger than your excuses. That strength carries over into every area of your life whether it's handling stress at work, navigating a tough relationship, or chasing a big goal, you'll find yourself thinking, *If I can do that, I can do this.*

THE CONNECTION BETWEEN MINDSET AND MOVEMENT

Each pillar in the SHIFTS Framework is connected to the others, working together to create lifelong fitness and wellness—but the connection between the Fitness pillar and the Thoughts and Mindset pillar is especially strong. I've seen one strengthen and benefit the other, and vice versa, over and over again in my life and in the lives of my clients.

Fitness has been an outlet to help me deal with anxiety, something I've struggled with since I was a painfully shy young girl. Being an athlete comes with a certain amount of pressure, and I've always had really high expectations of myself. Performance anxiety was a real challenge for me, but physical movement and good nutrition helped. You know what else helped? Knowing I wasn't the only one who dealt with it.

I remember hearing Dolly Parton share something in an interview before a performance. She said something like "I always get nervous before a performance, but that's because I care. If you don't get nervous, it probably doesn't mean that much to you." Hearing that reminded me that performance anxiety is normal, and if Dolly can push through, so can I.

As a child and a young woman, fitness helped me overcome my shyness. My background as a professional dancer, competitive gymnast, and competitive and professional cheerleader taught me how to thrive under pressure while also staying composed, focused, disciplined, and grounded in the spotlight. This lesson was even more important for me to honor behind the scenes when no one was watching. But when I started competing in CrossFit, the performance anxiety came back stronger than ever. Not only did I get anxious before competitions, I started experiencing anxiety before workouts, even if I wasn't competing. I used all the energy I needed for the workout worrying how the workout would go.

It was hard, but I knew I needed to face my anxiety head-on. I took my training intensity down a notch and shifted my focus to powerlifting and functional gymnastics only for a time. I learned how to coach myself through anxious moments and keep going. I also learned how to focus on the constants in my life, one of which was the SHIFTS Framework. I found that if I stuck to a plan and stayed consistent in training, nutrition, and daily lifestyle habits—controlling what was within my power to control and letting the rest go—I was able to lower the anxiety and make it manageable consistently. One of the things that helped the most was learning how to release pressure and manage my expectations, which is what I want to talk about next.

RELEASING PRESSURE AND MANAGING EXPECTATIONS

I've always been someone who sets high standards for myself, and while that can be a strength, it can also create unnecessary stress. I'd walk into the gym expecting to crush every workout, to push myself harder than the day before each and every day. But that mindset wasn't sustainable. It was exhausting.

Thankfully, I've learned how to pace myself and approach each session with an open mind. Some days, I'm ready to go all in even if I know it will be hard. Other days, I might just need to get training in without pushing myself to my max. I give myself grace and allow myself to complete the workout at whatever pace I need to that day without worrying about speed or intensity.

And you know what? When I take the pressure off, I often find I can go faster or lift heavier than I expected. The same has been true for my clients, and I talk with them about this often. When you release those rigid expectations, you discover your true capacity. Facing something difficult like anxiety is never fun, but you can confront challenges head-on and not let them stand in your way.

Reframing how you think about your fitness can really make a difference in your overall health and wellness, too. Research shows that the way we talk about physical activity really matters. In a study conducted from 2016 to 2019, college students who were given exercise guidelines that suggested a smaller amount of activity and a more flexible idea of what "counts" as exercise felt like what they were doing was valuable, and that mindset made a big difference.[1]

Instead of feeling overwhelmed or like they weren't measuring up, participants felt more confident, stayed more active, and even reported feeling healthier just one week later. The takeaway? Setting realistic and approachable goals can actually motivate people to move more and feel better about their progress. It's a great reminder that small steps and feeling like "enough" can lead to big results.

But what makes mindset growth possible? How is it that we can train our brains? It all boils down to neuroplasticity.

NEUROPLASTICITY

Here's something I wish people knew more about: The human brain is *incredibly* adaptable. That is thanks to a little thing called neuroplasticity—your brain's built-in ability to change, rewire, and grow based on what you do, think, and experience.[2] It's how we learn new skills, break old habits, create new habits, and bounce back from challenges. And when it comes to training your mindset right alongside your body? Neuroplasticity is your secret weapon.

There are two main types of neuroplasticity. The first type is structural plasticity. This refers to the brain's ability to physically change its structure in response to learning or experience. The second type is functional plasticity, which refers to the brain's ability to shift functions from damaged areas to healthy areas after injury.

Every time you push through a tough workout, choose a growth mindset instead of frustration, or remind yourself that you *can* do hard things—you're not only building muscle. You're literally reshaping your brain. You're training it to respond with resilience, focus, and confidence.[3]

This is especially important when you're leveling up your fitness. Because the mental side? It's just as demanding as the physical. You're going to hit moments where your body says, "Nope," and your mind gets loud with doubt. That's when neuroplasticity will kick in if you let it. With consistent effort, you can create new mental patterns that support your goals instead of sabotaging them.

So the next time you catch yourself saying, "I'm just not good at this," stop and reframe. Say, "I'm not good at it *yet.*" That little shift is neuroplasticity in action—and it's how lifelong strength, health, and happiness are built.

Not every workout has to be your best. Not every session needs to break records. Some days, just showing up is enough. Without the mental pressure weighing you down, you can focus on the process instead of the outcome. Remind yourself to just start and do what you can, *one rep, one movement, one step, and one day at a time.*

What I love most about fitness is how it trains your mind as much as your body. Every workout is an opportunity to practice resilience, to get comfortable being uncomfortable, and to rewrite any narrative in your head. When you're in the middle of a tough workout and everything in you wants to stop, that's when you have an opportunity to build mental strength. You learn how to quiet the doubts, focus on your breath, and take it one movement at a time.

This mental training doesn't just help in the gym—it spills over into every aspect of life. When anxiety creeps in during other situations, I remind myself of what I've learned in those workouts. I mentally tell myself, *I've been here before. I've faced hard things and gotten through them. I can do it again.* That simple mindset shift has helped me handle stress, navigate challenges, and stay grounded in moments of uncertainty.

When I look back on my own journey, the moments that stand out the most aren't the ones where things came easily. They're the times when I doubted myself, felt overwhelmed, or wanted to quit and chose to keep going anyway. Those were the moments that taught me what I'm truly capable of, and those are lessons I try to pass on to every client I work with.

You are capable of more than you think. When you learn to shift your mindset, to replace fear with curiosity, and to take consistent action—even when it's hard—you'll start to see those limits fall away. Once you realize what you're capable of, there's no going back. You'll carry that strength with you into every part of your life.

Start today. Take one small step toward the life you want to create. Maybe it's showing up for a workout, taking five minutes to quiet your mind, or simply replacing one negative thought with a positive one. Whatever it is, know that every small effort counts. Every step forward, no matter how tiny, is actually a step toward building a stronger, healthier, and happier life.

I can promise you that this journey is worth all of the effort you'll put in along the way. When you take control of your mind and your actions, you're not just building strength for today. You're building strength for tomorrow and the rest of your life.

KEY TAKEAWAYS FOR SECTION 7.5

1. **Mindset matters.** You can do everything right physically, but if your thoughts aren't aligned, progress will stall.
2. **Coach yourself, don't criticize.** Your inner voice is powerful. Make it work for you, not against you. Flip the script when doubt shows up.
3. **Mental strength is built in the hard stuff.** Growth happens when your mind carries you through challenges.

4. **Pick one empowering thought.** Keep it simple. Choose a mantra and repeat it when things get tough.
5. **You can rewire your brain.** Mindset isn't fixed. Every better thought is a rep toward a stronger response.

[1] Octavia H. Zahrt and Alia J. Crum, "Effects of Physical Activity Recommendations on Mindset, Behavior and Perceived Health," *Preventive Medicine Reports* 17 (2019): 101027, https://doi.org/10.1016/j.pmedr.2019.101027.
[2] Norman Doidge, *The Brain That Changes Itself: Stories of Personal Triumph from the Frontiers of Brain Science* (New York: Viking, 2007).
[3] Bryan Kolb and Ian Q. Whishaw, "Brain Plasticity and Behavior," *Annual Review of Psychology* 49 (1998): 43–64, https://doi.org/10.1146/annurev.psych.49.1.43.

SECTION 7.6: SUNSHINE

If I sat down and made a list of my favorite things to do, most of them would include lots of fresh air and sunshine. Even as a kid, I spent more time outside than inside engaged in activities like surfing, swimming, boating and fishing, jet skiing, tubing, biking, and gardening with my family. Today, I'm blessed to live in San Diego, one of the sunniest places in the country, so things haven't changed that much. On any given day, you're likely to find me outdoors or on the water fishing, swimming, boating, surfing, or paddleboarding. Other days, it's biking through town, browsing a farmers market, hitting the trails for a hike, or finding a moment of calm with some yoga or a beach run. I live for moments on or near the water, in the wild, or anywhere that fuels my movement and joy. There's nothing quite like being outside in the sunshine to make me feel like all is right with the world.

And it turns out, there's a good reason for that. Sunshine isn't just something that feels good—it's something that's essential for our health and well-being. In fact, sunshine is the final pillar of my SHIFTS Framework because of its incredible impact on both our bodies and minds.

SUNLIGHT'S HISTORY AS A NATURAL HEALER

Did you know that for centuries, sunlight has been recognized for its therapeutic effects in combating diseases like rickets and tuberculosis (TB)? The connection between sunlight and these conditions highlights the essential role of vitamin D and ultraviolet (UV) light in promoting healing and overall health.

Rickets is a condition characterized by soft, weak bones, and it's commonly caused by a vitamin D deficiency. Vitamin D helps the body absorb calcium and phosphorus, which are essential nutrients that build strong bones. In the early 20th century, researchers observed that children living in industrial cities with limited sunlight exposure were more likely to develop rickets.[5] When they exposed children to sunlight, it significantly improved their symptoms by boosting their vitamin D levels. Eventually, foods like milk were fortified with vitamin D to prevent rickets and TB. Before antibiotics were discovered, sunlight therapy was one of the main treatments for TB.[7]

As a bonus, sunlight was found to stimulate the immune system, improve lung function, and accelerate wound healing in those with skin manifestations of TB.[6] UV rays were thought to kill bacteria directly while also enhancing the production of vitamin D, which played a role in immune defense.

Recent research has confirmed these historical observations. Vitamin D, synthesized in the skin through sunlight exposure, helps balance the immune system, making it more effective in fighting TB bacteria. A study by Nnoaham and Clarke from 2008 revealed that vitamin D deficiency is associated with an increased risk of TB, supporting the long-standing connection between sunlight and TB recovery.[7]

While medical advancements like antibiotics and supplements have largely replaced sunlight therapy, these lessons from history remind us of sunlight's powerful role in human health. For people with conditions like rickets or

TB, sunlight exposure combined with modern treatment continues to be an essential tool for prevention and recovery.

THE SCIENCE BEHIND SUNSHINE

Did you know that just 15–20 minutes of direct sunlight on exposed skin each day can do wonders for your health? It's so simple that it's easily overlooked, but the sun provides something we struggle to get enough of anywhere else—vitamin D. This powerful nutrient also plays a crucial role in many bodily functions, like calcium absorption to support strong bones and prevent conditions like osteoporosis. It also helps with mood regulation, which assists in preventing depression and lessening anxiety. Plus, vitamin D provides immune system support to keep your body strong and resilient.[2]

In fact, vitamin D is so important that a single half-hour in the summer sun can trigger the release of tens of thousands of International Units (IU) of vitamin D in your body, depending on your skin tone. If you're fair-skinned, sunshine produces 50,000 IU of vitamin D that can be absorbed, while tanned or darker-skinned people absorb slightly less due to the protective effect of melanin.[1]

Beyond vitamin D, sunlight also plays a key role in regulating your body's circadian rhythms, or the natural sleep-wake cycle that controls your energy levels, metabolism, and mental clarity. Exposing your eyes to sunlight first thing in the morning helps signal to your brain that it's time to wake up. This can boost your energy and mood for the day ahead. Neuroscientists like Andrew Huberman have highlighted how morning sunlight is a simple yet powerful habit to improve overall health.[3] But don't stress if mornings are chaotic or begin well before the sunlight. Getting sunlight at any point during the day still provides incredible benefits.

WHY SUNSHINE MATTERS FOR MENTAL HEALTH

The connection between sunlight and mental health is strong. Have you ever noticed how being outside in the sun instantly lifts your spirits? That's because sunlight triggers the release of serotonin, a hormone that boosts your mood and helps you feel calm and focused. This is why spending time in the sun can be especially helpful during the winter months when shorter days and limited sunlight can lead to seasonal affective disorder (SAD).[4]

If you live in an area with limited sunshine, especially in the colder, darker months with less natural light, you might consider getting a sun lamp that simulates natural light and can help keep serotonin levels balanced.

For me, sunshine has always been a form of therapy. After I had my daughter, those early postpartum weeks were some of the most mentally and emotionally challenging of my life. I vividly remember how transformative it was to step outside even for just 15 minutes. Standing in the sunshine, feeling the warmth on my skin, and breathing in fresh air was like hitting the reset button. It reminded me that I was still me. I was still connected to the world outside of sleepless nights and diaper changes. That small, simple act of stepping outside helped me feel more grounded and gave me the strength to keep going.

A NATURAL MOOD BOOSTER

Sunshine is one of those simple, often overlooked, elements of a healthy lifestyle. It's free and available in most parts of the world. That can make it easy to take it for granted. When you start being intentional about soaking in those rays though, you'll notice a difference in your mood, energy, and overall well-being. Whether you're feeling overwhelmed, stressed, or just stuck, stepping outside for even a few minutes can shift your perspective and help you reconnect with yourself.

Sunshine is more thana feel good experience. It's a cornerstone of health. From boosting your mood to regulating your body's rhythms and providing essential vitamin D, sunlight is a gift that supports every part of your well-being. So, let's keep it simple. Take a moment to step outside, feel the warmth on your skin, and let nature do its magic.

You deserve it.

Sunshine is also a great pillar to pair up with one of the other pillars. You can grab lunch and hydrate in the sunshine, do an outdoor workout, do mindset work outside in the sun, or even catch a quick cat nap in a sunny spot.

As we bring chapter 7 to a close, I've given you my prescription of tools that will offer you lifelong fitness and wellness. Sunshine mixed with a good night's sleep, delicious whole foods, lots of water, intense bursts of fitness followed by active recovery sessions, rest days, and quiet time will all yield so much more in return than what you invest.

In the next chapter, I'm going to cover a couple more things that will help you along your health journey. Then in

Part 3 of this book, I'll share how to assess and track your fitness and wellness. Finally, I'll share my best, easy-to-implement tips for all six pillars of my SHIFTS formula, so you can choose one or two to start and layer together to create the elements I ask you to build so that you can engage in new, healthy habits—one step at a time.

KEY TAKEAWAYS FOR SECTION 7.6

1. **Sunshine is free medicine.** Just 15 to 20 minutes a day in the sun boosts mood, sleep, immunity, and vitamin D—no pills needed.
2. **Get outside.** Fresh air and sunlight can lift your mindset and help you feel more grounded.
3. **Light supports energy and sleep.** Daily sun exposure helps regulate your rhythm, improve your bone health, and protect your mental health.
4. **Stack your habits.** Walk, hydrate, journal, or stretch in the sun. Layering healthy habits adds momentum.
5. **Make it part of your day.** Take a short walk, sit by a window, or try a sun lamp in low-light seasons.
6. **Let nature reset you.** Sunshine reminds you to slow down, breathe, and reconnect with the bigger picture of life.

[1] Michael Nathaniel Mead, "Benefits of Sunlight: A Bright Spot for Human Health," *Environmental Health Perspectives* 116, no. 4 (2008): A160–A167, https://doi.org/10.1289/ehp.116-a160.

[2] Michael F. olick, "Sunlight and Vitamin D for Bone Health and Prevention of Autoimmune Diseases, Cancers, and Cardiovascular Disease." *The American Journal of Clinical Nutrition* 80, no. 6 (2004): 1678S–1688S. https://academic. oup.com/ajcn/article/80/6/1678S/4690460.

[3] Andrew Huberman, "The Science of Morning Sunlight for Health and Sleep," *The Huberman Lab Podcast*, accessed Jan 2025, https://hubermanlab.com/.

[4] Arthur Ecker, "Reflex Sympathetic Dystrophy Thermography in Diagnosis: Psychiatric Considerations." *Psychiatric Annals*. 1984;14(11):787-793. doi:10.3928/0048-5713-19841101-08.

[5] Alfred F. Hess and Lester J. Unger, "The Cure of Infantile Rickets by Artificial Light and Sunlight," *Proceedings of the Society for Experimental Biology and Medicine* 18, no. 1 (1921): 298–299.

[6] Auguste Rollier, "Heliotherapy in Lupus Vulgaris and Pulmonary Tuberculosis," *The Lancet* 214, no. 5543 (1929): 931–933.

[7] Kelechi E. Nnoaham and Aileen Clarke, 2008, "Low Serum Vitamin D Levels and Tuberculosis: A Systematic Review and Meta-Analysis," *International Journal of Epidemiology* 37 (1): 113–119. https://doi.org/10.1093/ije/dym247.

Chapter 8
Infectious Positive Influences

I've always been a pretty self-motivated person. From a young age, I had this deep desire to push myself, to see what I was capable of, and to constantly improve. Whether it was gymnastics, cheerleading and dance, or training on my own, I was used to working hard, setting goals, and figuring things out without much help. I used my training time as a form of a quiet time with myself, and if you'd have asked me if I was looking for more community in my life, I'd have told you I was good just doing my own thing.

That changed the first time I stepped into a CrossFit gym. I wasn't familiar with the community aspect of CrossFit, and until then, I'd never realized how powerful it was to have people around me who genuinely want to see me win. I remember being in the middle of a workout with lungs burning, muscles shaking, and every part of me wanting to stop…but then I heard voices cheering me on, pushing me to keep going. And it wasn't just the coach! Other people in the class, some of whom I barely even knew, had paused in their own workout to encourage and hype me up. It was a different kind of energy, and it was infectious.

Who you surround yourself with matters.

You can be the most driven person in the world, but if you're constantly surrounded by negativity, doubt, or people who don't challenge you to be better, it's going to be a lot harder to reach your full potential. On the other hand, if you intentionally place yourself in environments where people uplift, encourage, and push you beyond what you thought you were capable of, whether that's in fitness, business, or life, you'll start to see massive growth.

The truth is, success isn't only about talent, hard work, or luck. It's about the habits you build, the energy you allow into your life, and the people you choose to be around. When you surround yourself with the right people, their energy, discipline, and mindset will start to rub off on you.

This chapter is all about how to cultivate those infectious positive influences that will help you as you implement the SHIFTS Framework in your own life. It's about setting yourself up for success by choosing supportive environments, effective habits, and people who fit and align with your goals, values, and vision. Whether you're just starting out on your fitness journey, working toward a personal goal, or looking to level up in any area of your life, the principles in this chapter will help you build a support system that fuels your growth and pushes you to become your best self.

You don't have to do it alone. And in fact, you'll go so much further with the SHIFTS Framework when you have support. So, let's dive in.

COMMUNITY AND CONNECTION

I was pleasantly surprised from the very first CrossFit workout I did in a group class. The setting was so different. I had never received coaching in that way before— where someone helped me with my form, technique, and gave me real-time feedback (outside of sport-specific training I had for gymnastics, cheer, and dance).

During that workout, I was doing something that felt like the hardest thing I'd ever done in my life as far as physical fitness went. And the coach was right there, saying, "You're doing awesome," breaking down the high volume of reps into manageable chunks with a verbal countdown, "Take a breath. Okay, 5, 4, 3, 2, 1—go." It was like I suddenly had a support system I didn't even know I needed.

After the workout, everyone was completely spent and lying on the floor. Yet we were also cheering each other on, high-fiving each other from the floor, and encouraging those still working. It didn't matter if you were a beginner or advanced. Everyone was there showing up for themselves and supporting others. I never thought I needed people cheering me on or high-fiving me. But being surrounded by like-minded people who were working hard and showing up for their health and quality of life felt completely different from anything I'd experienced before.

No matter how self-motivated you are, surrounding yourself with like-minded people makes all the difference. The energy of a group, the accountability of a community, and the support of people who genuinely want you to succeed can push you to new levels you never thought possible.

That's the power of community, something I firmly believe everyone needs. You might be familiar with the quote, "You are the average of the five people you spend the most time with." I've heard this saying so many times, and the more I experience life, the more I see how true it is.

The people you surround yourself with influence your mindset, habits, and attitude. If you're constantly around people who complain, make excuses, or don't prioritize their health, it becomes that much harder to stay committed to your goals. But if you're around people who push themselves, challenge their limits, and show up with a positive attitude—that energy rubs off on you. They're infectious positive influences, right?

Think about the people in your life right now. Are they lifting you up or holding you back? Are they inspiring you to be better or making you feel like your goals are too big?

If you want to level up your fitness and wellness, you need to intentionally place yourself in environments that support growth. Join a gym where people push and encourage each other. Ask around to see which locations local friends and family members recommend. Seek out a coach or trainer who challenges you to think bigger. Surround yourself with people who align with the type of life you want to create.

The truth is, you can't expect to thrive in a negative environment. If you want to elevate your lifelong fitness and wellness, you have to surround yourself with people who are already living at that level. Next, let's take a look at the amazing concepts a positive community can support you with.

Accountability

One of the biggest benefits of community is accountability. When you're training alone, it might be easier to skip a workout or take it easy when you don't feel like pushing yourself. But when you're part of a group, you're way more likely to stay consistent.

There will be days you don't feel like working out. There will be workouts you'll be tempted to quit halfway through. On your own, it's much easier to give in to that feeling. But with people around you, encouraging you, and holding you to a higher standard, you're much more likely to push through. And every time you do, you'll walk away mentally and physically stronger.

The same goes for my clients. The ones who have a strong support system—whether it's their family, a spouse, a parent or child, or an accountability partner—are the ones who stay consistent and see the best results. They don't just rely on motivation; they rely on the people around them to keep them accountable and help them keep showing up. I do want to say, though, that accountability does *not* mean comparing yourself to others in a negative way.

Breaking the Comparison Trap

One of the most surprising things I learned from training in a community setting was how it changed my relationships. Something shifted when I became part of a supportive fitness community like CrossFit where we cheered for and encouraged each other. Instead of looking at others and thinking, "I'm not as good as them," I thought, "Wow, look at what's possible." I have always been inspired by what others who have gone before me were able to accomplish. Their success wasn't a threat—it was inspiration for my goals and proof that I could push myself to a higher level, too.

The same can apply to your fitness and wellness journey. When you surround yourself with people who are winning, it shouldn't make you feel like you're behind. It can show you what's possible. Let your community remind you that you're capable of more than you think, and that with a strong mindset and the right support system, you can achieve anything.

A supportive community will push you, challenge you, and remind you why you started on the days you feel like giving up. So, if you're not already surrounded by people who inspire you—go find them. Surround yourself with friends who push you to be better. Seek out mentors who will help you think bigger. And as you grow, don't forget that you can also be that kind of person for someone else.

Surrounding yourself with infectious positive influences— whether that's people cheering you on or showing you which habits will take you to the next level—can completely transform your mindset, motivation, and success. Finding a supportive community can help you reach goals you never thought possible.

As I close out Part 2 of this book, I want you to know that you should be *so* proud of yourself! You're building a strong foundation for your fitness and wellness journey by learning about all six pillars in my SHIFTS Framework, and that's something to celebrate.

Now, the only thing left is to start taking action, and Part 3 of this book makes doing that simple and straightforward. In chapter 9, you'll learn how to assess your starting point, and in chapter 10, I'll give you my downloadable tracker and show you how to use it. Finally, chapter 11 contains my best tips for applying all six pillars in the SHIFTS Framework in your day-to-day life so you can create real, lasting results.

KEY TAKEAWAYS FOR CHAPTER 8

1. **Your circle matters.** The people around you shape your mindset. Choose those who help you grow, show up to keep you accountable, and cheer you on when you're attempting something difficult.
2. **Community fuels consistency.** When motivation dips, accountability and support keep you going.
3. **Surround yourself wisely.** Not everyone will get your goals, and that's okay. Find those who do, and build an environment that supports your growth.

PART 3

**Putting the SHIFTS
Framework to Work**

Chapter 9

Laying the Foundation

Clarity fuels momentum. If you want to start off strong and set yourself up for success, before anything else, get clear and ground yourself in your "why" for starting my SHIFTS Framework.

With every new fitness client I work with, we first determine their "why." Each client fills out a Health and Fitness Questionnaire, which helps me decide where to start with their individualized plan. One of the questions is "What are your health and fitness goals for the next year? Next three years? Next five years?" Everyone's answers are unique to their lives and their desires. Here are a few answers I've received:

I want to increase my knowledge and strength in bodyweight movements. Ready to compete in 2019 Granite Games. In three years, I'd like to have a sub-20 minute 5K, power clean 500 pounds, squat 350 pounds, string five muscle-ups together. In five years, I want to find my peak fitness level and have a plan to maintain it for the rest of my life.

I want to remain healthy, strong, and lean. The same for the next three to five years. Learn and master new movements like bar muscle-up and butterfly pull-ups.

I want great health, then greater health. A six-pack, lose all excess fat, be stronger, gain some muscle, and become much more flexible. Goal to be able to do the splits by next summer.

My nutrition sucks because I'm not very good at cooking. I want to eat healthier and be educated on food— including macros and protein intake.

I want to train like a bodybuilder and eventually compete. Overall, I just want to continue to build my strength while staying lean. I also want a big booty, LOL.

I feel so much better when I'm toned with muscle—from my core to my legs. I really need to course correct my posture before it's too late. I don't love having huge arm muscles, but I am open to getting toned and feeling strong. Fitness has been a part of my life for years, so I really am looking for a level set and to rebuild muscles, tone, and feel great for my wedding. After that, I'd like to maintain everything and focus on prenatal efforts for building a family. I'd like to also stay strong/work out during this next chapter of my life. I know I will have to focus on PT-related items for my hip labrum as well.

Every single one of those answers has the power to help them stay motivated, consistent and moving with forward momentum once they start. Setting your "why" as you begin is so important. Now it's your turn. Write your answer in the space below or in a notebook or journal.

> **What are your health and fitness goals for the next year? Next three years? Next five years? Why (So you can…)?**

Want to see the rest of the Health and Fitness Questionnaire? You can download it from the Book Resources section of my website. It's a great resource for you—and also for your coach or trainer if you choose to work with one.

SET REALISTIC EXPECTATIONS

Once you've set your "why," it's time to set realistic expectations—and *realistic* is the key word here. One of the fastest ways to burn out in fitness, business, or life is by starting off with completely unrealistic expectations. I've seen it happen so many times. Someone decides they're finally going to commit to getting in shape, so they go all in. They're working out six days a week, cutting out all their favorite foods, and expecting to see results overnight. Guess what happens? Two weeks later they're exhausted, frustrated, and ready to quit.

I get it. When you're motivated, you want results *now*. You want to feel stronger, look better, and prove to yourself that you can do it. And progress is relative. A small accomplishment for one person might be far too big for another person to attempt until they're further along in their progress. The truth is, real progress takes time. And if you expect instant results, you're setting yourself up for disappointment. Small, consistent actions always beat extreme, unsustainable efforts.

THE POWER OF HABIT STACKING

One of the best ways to set yourself up for long-term success to achieve your goals is by habit stacking. Habit stacking is the idea that you'll experience less resistance to creating a new habit if you attach the new habit to one your brain is already used to. This is a concept I learned in a multi-level coaching certification and from author James Clear. Here's how it works in four simple steps:

Step 1: Identify something you already do well. For example, let's say you always take a multivitamin first thing in the morning. What's something from the SHIFTS formula you could add to that existing habit? How about drinking a full glass of water with the multivitamin?

Step 2: Track your progress for two to three weeks. I provide a downloadable tracker in chapter 10 that you can use.

Step 3: Notice when this new habit becomes part of your daily routine.

Step 4: Choose another healthy habit from the SHIFTS Framework. Link it to another existing habit and keep stacking!

Instead of trying to overhaul your entire life in one day, focus on one key action at a time. Layer on new habits and build on them mindfully over days, weeks, and months. If you're new to working out, instead of starting with a six-day workout plan, start with two or three days a week and build from there so your body has time to adjust and recover.

In the same way, if you want to improve your nutrition, start with a simple change, like drinking more water or eating more protein with each meal. Small changes lead to big results over time. By leading with small changes, you're setting yourself up to win with things you can follow through on. Start small and stay consistent, and before you know it, you'll be making huge progress without even realizing it.

Record the simple change you'll start with by checking the pillar and writing the specific action you'll take in the space below, or add it to your notebook or journal. If the simple change could easily be paired with another simple change from another pillar, you can write more than one...but remember, keep your goals realistic. I've included an example below.

EXAMPLE: Check the pillar(s) from the SHIFTS Framework you will start with and write the specific action(s) you'll take in the space below.

Sleep _____

Hydration I will replace one cup of coffee with a glass of water per day.

Intake _____

Fitness _____

Thoughts _____

Sunshine I will drink one glass of water outside each day.

Now it's your turn:

Check the pillar(s) from the SHIFTS Framework you will start with and write the specific action(s) you'll take in the space below.

Sleep _____

Hydration _____

Intake _____

Fitness _____

Thoughts _____

Sunshine _____

FOCUS ON PROGRESS, NOT PERFECTION

There's one more important thing about progress that can really mess with setting realistic expectations. And that's the false idea that you aren't making progress if everything you do isn't perfect. I can't tell you how many times I've seen people give up just because they didn't do something perfectly. They miss one workout, eat one unhealthy meal, or have one bad day and suddenly they feel like they've failed. But let me tell you something—you don't have to be perfect to make progress.

Your success isn't determined by one meal, one workout, or even one week. It's determined by what you do consistently over time. The people who reach their goals aren't the ones who never mess up. They're the ones who keep going even if they do.

Instead of expecting perfection, focus on making progress. Setbacks will happen. You'll have days where you don't feel like doing the work. Just keep showing up. That's what leads to real, lasting change. In Part 3 of this book, I'll show you how to track your progress to help you stay accountable—and encouraged—as you see yourself progress.

TRUST THE PROCESS

A final word on starting strong by setting expectations—it's important to allow yourself to trust the process. When I was training as a gymnast, I had to learn patience. Skills that seemed impossible at first eventually became second nature, not because I mastered them overnight, but because I showed up and put in the reps, day after day.

We broke each skill down into little tiny movements called progressions or drills. Then we worked those drills over and over again, perfecting body position, timing, technique, and confidence.

After training and perfecting each movement individually, we attempted bigger chunks of the specific skill we were working toward. Finally, we put it all together to achieve the full skill. If you want to see an example of how this works, visit the Resources section of this book to learn how to access the Body Movement Appendix, where you can find written, photo, and video breakdowns of movements and progressions.

The body and the mind work together over a period of time to develop a ton of muscle memory. You gain a level of confidence and familiarity with moving your body through specific shapes and positions at a certain speed until eventually you master the skill. The same applies to any skill you work toward.

Give yourself time to grow, and be kind to yourself along the way. Focus on consistency, celebrate the small wins, and give yourself the grace to keep going no matter how long it takes. If you stay committed to the process, the results will come, along with many other amazing perks along the way, like increased stamina and more confidence and self-esteem!

KEY TAKEAWAYS FOR CHAPTER 9

1. **Start now.** There's no perfect time—begin where you are with what you have.
2. **Build slowly.** Start with one to two workouts a week and add light movement on other days. Keep your plans sustainable.
3. **Make it fit you.** Choose a routine that works with your life—not someone else's.
4. **Know your "why."** Your deeper reason for moving forward with your goals will keep you going when things get tough.
5. **Progress takes time.** Stay patient, trust the process, and celebrate small wins along the way.

Chapter 10
Tracking Your Progress

*I*f you don't track your fitness and wellness, how do you really know where you stand?

That's a question I ask my clients. We think we're eating enough protein, drinking enough water, and getting enough sleep, but when we actually start tracking the data, the numbers might tell a different story. One of the most important things you can do for yourself starting right now, today, is to begin tracking your fitness and wellness behaviors.

What gets measured gets managed. If you've ever felt like you're doing all the right things but not seeing progress, tracking will show you exactly where the gaps are. You may find you're getting five hours of sleep instead of the six or seven you thought. You may realize your hydration is inconsistent or that you're missing protein targets by more than you realized. Once you see the patterns, you can start making adjustments that actually move you forward—but it's hard to see the patterns if you don't measure what is really going on.

When you track your habits, you start to see how everything connects. You'll notice how your energy dips when you don't sleep well, how your workouts feel better when you're properly fueled, and how hydration impacts your focus. Tracking helps you take control of your choices instead of just reacting to how you feel in the moment.

And don't worry. You don't have to track forever. Think of it as a reset. Doing a short-term lifestyle audit—whether it's for a week, a month, or a season—gives you a reality check and helps you realign with your goals. Even if you've been consistent for years, tracking two to three times a year— something I have my clients do—can be a great way to check in and make sure you're in line with your goals.

I start all my fitness clients out with a lifestyle audit as a way to get them used to tracking their progress, and that's what I want you to start out doing, too. In this chapter, I'm going to give you some resources you can use to track your lifestyle habits so that you know where you stand. When you see what's really happening with your sleep, hydration, intake, fitness, thoughts, and sunshine, you're giving yourself the gift of information that will help you make the simple, intentional changes that lead to real results. You're no longer guessing—you're collecting data on your own life, and that data is powerful.

You don't have to track everything at once. Start with one or two areas—I recommend starting with sleep. Then, after a couple weeks add protein intake and water consumption. The goal isn't to be perfect. The goal is to create awareness, make small improvements, and build the strongest, healthiest, happiest version of yourself—one intentional step at a time.

STEP 1: ASSESS YOURSELF

If you're new to tracking, starting with a self-assessment is a great way to become aware of where you stand before making any changes. Remember the Health and Fitness Questionnaire I mentioned in the previous chapter? Time to fill one out for yourself! You can download it from the Book Resources section of my website (check the Resources section of this book for instructions on where to find it).

Use the Health and Fitness Questionnaire as your starting point. It will help you become aware of your daily lifestyle habits, understand where you are right now, and identify the areas you want to start with that will help you get to your goals. The questionnaire will ask you about your current training and your training intensity level. It will also ask you about your health concerns, nutrition, short- and long-term goals, sleep, and more.

I recommend you download the questionnaire, then print it out so you can record your information with pen and paper. There's something powerful about taking time to thoughtfully reflect on where you are and where you want to go, then physically writing the words out. Once you've filled out the Health and Fitness Questionnaire, you're ready to start implementing changes, one or two at a time. Here are my recommendations for what to track first.

STEP 2: TRACK SLEEP, PROTEIN, AND WATER INTAKE

Once you've finished the Health and Fitness Questionnaire, there are three things I recommend you track at first—sleep, protein, and water intake. Start by paying attention to the following areas for two to three weeks:

> **Sleep:** Many people wear sleep deprivation around like a badge of honor, but it's nothing to be proud of. Not getting enough sleep affects your mental health, immune system, hormones, and recovery, and it can also have serious long-term effects later in life, including the increased risk for diseases like Alzheimer's, obesity, and diabetes. Plus, a lack of sleep puts more stress on your body and mind, making it harder to keep doing all the things you do every day.
>
> Track what time you go to bed, what time you wake up, and how many total hours of sleep you get per night. Then take a moment to ask yourself the following questions:
>
> > Am I getting enough sleep?
> >
> > Is it good-quality, uninterrupted sleep? Do I wake up feeling rested?
> >
> > Am I struggling to fall asleep or stay asleep?
>
> **Protein:** Write down how many grams you're eating each day. A good target is 1 to 1.5 grams per pound of body weight. Aim to get most of your protein through food, mainly lean meats. A protein shake is okay, but

quality whole foods like organic, grassfed, locally sourced protein is a better source.

Water: Track how many ounces of water you drink per day. Aim for half your body weight in ounces per day at minimum, or more if you're active.

Whether it's first thing in the morning or right before bed, find a consistent time to log your sleep, protein, and water intake for each day. To make tracking easier, I've included a downloadable SHIFTS Tracker on the Book Resources page of my website. Check the Resources section of this book for the link.

After two to three weeks, take a step back and look at your results. Where are you crushing it? Where do you need a little more focus? This is where real change happens—when you see the trends and make small, intentional shifts to improve. As you add in new SHIFTS every two to three weeks, just print off another copy of the tracker so you can monitor your progress.

In the next chapter, I'm going to give you fast, actionable tips for shifting gears in all six pillars of my SHIFTS Framework. Don't feel like you have to tackle them all at once. Any of these tips will help you build a stronger, healthier, happier life. So, choose one or two to focus on at a time.

KEY TAKEAWAYS FOR CHAPTER 10

1. **What gets measured gets managed.** Tracking reveals the truth behind your habits and helps you make real progress.
2. **Start small.** Track sleep, water, and protein to begin. Add more over time.
3. **Know your baseline.** Use the Health and Fitness Questionnaire to get honest about where you're starting.
4. **Use your avatar as a filter.** Ask: Do my actions align with the version of me I am becoming? (This can be based on the work we did in chapter 4.)
5. **Track for insight, not perfection.** One week of tracking can reveal powerful patterns—no judgment, just clarity.
6. **Look for patterns.** Awareness connects your habits to your results—and puts you back in control.

Chapter 11

Best Tips for Core SHIFTS

I created the SHIFTS Framework to give you a structured, sustainable way to build lifelong habits for your strongest, healthiest, happiest life. But, none of this works if you don't take action. In this chapter, I'm going to give you simple, actionable steps you can take to make these core SHIFTS a permanent part of your life. Like I said in the previous chapter, you don't have to overhaul everything at once. Instead, you're going to build habits that actually fit into your real life and that you can use to create momentum. After all, consistency beats perfection every single time.

The tips I share in this chapter are based on things I personally do and things I've seen work over and over again for my clients. These are practical, no-nonsense strategies that will help you feel better, move more freely, recover faster, and show up stronger in every area of your life.

As you read through these tips, remember that you're in control. You get to decide what works for you, what you start with, and how you build from there. I gave you the tools you need to start tracking your progress in the previous chapter. Now it's time to choose one of the pillars in the SHIFTS Framework and take action on your fitness and wellness.

Maybe sleep is your biggest struggle right now, or maybe you need to focus on hydration. Maybe your workouts are solid, but your recovery habits need work. Wherever you're starting from right now, you're going to walk away from this chapter with clear, doable steps to help you make real progress.

SLEEP TIPS: CREATING A NIGHTTIME ROUTINE

A solid nighttime routine is one of the most important tools for better sleep, recovery, and overall well-being. I know firsthand how easy it is to push sleep to the back burner by staying up too late, scrolling through your phone, or squeezing in one more thing on your to-do list. But the truth is, quality sleep doesn't just happen. It's something you have to be intentional about. It's time to create a nighttime routine!

A nighttime routine is all about creating simple, consistent habits that signal to your body and brain that it's time to wind down. Our bodies respond best when we have a predictable rhythm before sleep. Follow these steps to create a nighttime routine.

Set a Consistent Bedtime

Going to bed and waking up at the same time every day—even on weekends—helps regulate your circadian rhythm, which controls your sleep-wake cycle. When you keep a consistent bedtime, your body starts to recognize when it's time to power down at night so that you wake up feeling refreshed in the morning. Aim for at least six hours of sleep per night, but closer to seven or eight is even better.

Limit Caffeine and Screen Time

Are you sabotaging your sleep with things you do earlier in the day? Caffeine can stay in your system for hours, so try to cut off coffee and other stimulants by early afternoon. Eating too close to bedtime can also interfere with sleep, so aim to have your last meal and drink at least two hours before bed.

Blue light from screens can mess with melatonin production, making it harder to fall asleep. Set a goal to turn off your phone, computer, and TV at least 30 minutes before bed. An hour, or more, is even better.

Create a Relaxing Pre-Sleep Routine

An evening routine should be calming and help transition your body from the busyness of the day to restful sleep. Here are some things that are part of my pre-sleep routine:

- Taking a warm bath or shower to help me unwind and relax my muscles
- Dimming the lights and burning some soothing candles
- Reading or journaling on paper, not on a screen
- Meditation or deep breathing to slow down my thoughts

Your nighttime routine doesn't have to look exactly like this. Experiment and find what works for you, then do it consistently. Even little things like sipping herbal tea or listening to soft music can make a difference in helping your body associate these habits with winding down.

Optimize Your Sleep Environment

How's your sleep environment? Is your bedroom set up for sleep? A cool, dark, and quiet space helps signal to your brain that it's time to shut down. Here are some tips for a restful sleep environment:

- Keep the room cool. Between 60–67 degrees is ideal.
- Use blackout curtains to block out light.
- Try a weighted blanket if you struggle with relaxation.
- Use white noise or a fan if you're a light sleeper.
- Invest in a good-quality mattress and pillow.

Make Sleep a Priority

Life happens, and some nights won't go according to plan. That's okay. If you can stick to your nighttime routine at least 80% to 90% of the time, you'll start to feel the benefits in your energy, recovery, and overall well-being.

If you're struggling with sleep, take inventory of your habits. Are you getting enough? Is the quality of your sleep good? Do you fall asleep easily but wake up in the middle of the night? You should also pay attention to what your sleep habits look like when you're training. Getting in your fitness time earlier in the day can help your mind and body achieve a more restful state later in the day, allowing for much higher quality sleep. Some form of vigorous fitness earlier in the day can help you fall asleep at night, stay asleep, and overcome sleep anxiety.

When training happens later in the day or evening, sometimes it becomes more difficult to wind down at a reasonable bedtime. Training also raises your core temperature, which can also affect your sleep quality depending on what time of day you get your training in.

Tracking your sleep will really help. Pay attention to the patterns and make small adjustments where needed. For help tracking your sleep, head back to chapter 10 to download the tracker.

HYDRATION TIPS: GETTING YOUR WATER IN

In Section 7.2, I talked about how a person's body weight in pounds divided by two is the number of ounces of water they need per day. So if you weigh 120 pounds, you need to drink at least 60 ounces of water daily. If you're active, you'll need even more. Here's how I make getting my water in more manageable:

- Find a container that holds half your daily water amount. For example, if you need 96 ounces, get a 48 ounce bottle and refill it twice.
- Drink one whole bottle before lunch, refill it, then drink the second half in the afternoon and early evening. Try to finish your water at least two hours before bed to avoid having to run to the bathroom in the middle of the night.
- Give your hydration a kick start by drinking a big glass of water first thing in the morning. That way, you'll be starting your day strong!

INTAKE TIPS FOR SUSTAINABLE NUTRITION

Making changes to your nutrition can feel intimidating at first. I get it. Life is busy, and the last thing you want is to feel like eating healthy is just one more thing on your never-ending to-do list. That's why I'm a big believer in keeping things simple and having a plan for your meals. Meal planning is the best way to set yourself up for success. It also saves you time and money.

Meal prepping is hands-down one of the best ways to stay on track. It might sound like a hassle, but trust me, it will save you so much time, money, and stress during the week. Start by picking one day—maybe Sunday or whatever day you have the most downtime—and use it to plan and prep your meals. Here's how I like to do it:

Plan your meals: Write down what you want to eat for the week. Focus on simple meals with plenty of protein (fish, pork, steak, chicken), veggies, and healthy fats.

Batch cook staples: Grill or bake a bunch of chicken breasts, roast a big tray of veggies, cook up a pot of quinoa or sweet potatoes—whatever your go-to foods are.

Portion it out: Divide everything into containers so you have grab-and-go meals ready when you need them. That way, you're not stuck scrambling for food when you're busy.

When your fridge is stocked with prepped meals, it's so much easier to stick to your goals. Plus, it keeps you from relying on takeout or convenience foods, which often don't align with how you want to be eating.

I'm all about keeping things simple when it comes to nutrition. You don't need to cook fancy, complicated meals to eat well. The main emphasis should be on making sure you're getting enough of the main character, protein, plus the complex carbohydrates in whole food form in the right serving size. Focus on foods that are easy to prepare and nutrient dense. I recommend eating four to five times a day to keep your blood sugar balanced and energy levels stable. When I'm prepping for a show, I typically eat five to six ounces of protein with four to five ounces of complex carbs for each meal. Here's an example of what my meals look like when I'm not prepping for a show:

7:00 am (Breakfast): 5–6 ounces of protein paired with 4–5 ounces of complex carbs

Some solid breakfast food options that are low to no added sodium include egg whites, oats, berries, protein pancakes (made with egg whites, cottage cheese, oats, and cinnamon), grits, unsweetened Greek yogurt, protein granola, nuts, nut butter, and chia jam. If you're doing paleo, look for gluten-free options for grits and bread. I also really enjoy Dave's Killer Bread for treat meals when I'm not in prep mode. It's a good option with five grams of protein per slice, but it's not gluten free.

10:00 am (Snack): 5–6 ounces of protein paired with 4–5 ounces of complex carbs

1:00 pm (Lunch): 5–6 ounces of protein paired with 4–5 ounces of complex carbs

For my morning snack and lunch, I pack double the amount of protein and complex carbs, then eat half at 10:00 am and half at 1:00 pm.

4:00 pm (Snack): 5–6 ounces of protein paired with 4–5 ounces of complex carbs

7:00 pm (Dinner): 5–6 ounces of protein paired with 4–5 ounces of complex carbs

If I won't be near my kitchen between 4:00 pm and 7:00 pm, I pack double the amount of protein and complex carbs for my afternoon snack and dinner. Then I eat half at 4:00 pm and half at 7:00 pm.

Great protein options for snacks and meals include chicken, fish, and other lean meats. Sweet potatoes or regular potatoes, squash, brussels sprouts, green leafy vegetables, and berries are good complex carb options.

For example, good snack/meal combo would be:
- Grilled chicken, roasted Brussels sprouts, and avocado
- A big salad with mixed greens, steak, ½ tablespoon olive oil, and a handful of nuts
- Ground turkey with sautéed zucchini and sweet potato

Steer clear of fake sweeteners. If you need something sweet, sometimes it's healthier for you to just enjoy the real thing in moderation during a treat meal.

Finally, and most importantly, remember to give yourself grace. Nutrition is a journey, not a destination. You don't have to be perfect to make progress. Some weeks will be better than others, and that's okay. What matters is that you're showing up for yourself and making choices that align with your goals most of the time.

FITNESS TIPS: CORE BODYWEIGHT FOUNDATIONS

There are two foundational static holds—body positions that require you to use your muscles to keep you strong and connected from head to toe—that I start my clients out with. These positions engage a good majority, if not all, of the body's muscles and are the starting point for all movement. One of the best things you can do as you start your fitness and wellness journey is to master these two positions by using static holds.

Hollow Body Position

Refined skill is not something you discover. It is built one day, one session, and one movement at a time. The hollow body position is one of the most foundational body positions for total body strength and body awareness. In gymnastics, we use it to teach control and proper alignment, but it's a position that applies to almost every movement you'll encounter in fitness. This position is one of my favorites because it enforces the importance of consistency, self-discipline, patience, focus, and process. One thing must follow the other, and at no point can you abandon your roots or your fundamentals.

Hollow body position enables the body to act as one big, solid piece of muscle. To achieve that effect, you must engage the entire body from your fingertips all the way down through your toes.

The Standard for Hollow Body Position:

1. Lie down on your back on the floor and work on extending your arms overhead while hugging your arms to your ears. Compress your ribs towards your hips.
2. Keep your shoulder blades elevated above the floor, your ribs tucked towards your hips, and your belly button pulled towards your spine.
3. Tuck your tailbone.
4. Squeeze your glutes—the muscles in your rear end—hard, straighten your legs, making sure to squeeze and fully engage your quads. Make sure your heels stay together and elevated with your toes pointed.

Why point your toes? Pointing your toes is not just for aesthetics. It keeps the rest of your body in check. If you have "dead fish feet" hanging off the end of your legs, chances are you're not as tight as you should be. Always remember to point and squeeze!

Want to see hollow body position in action? Check out the video demonstration in the Book Resources section of my website. You can find the link in the Resources section of this book.

Tight Arch Position

The tight arch, or "Superman" position, complements the

hollow body position. This movement strengthens your entire posterior chain—the group of muscles that run along the back side of your body from your neck down to your heels—which includes everything from your calves to your hamstrings, glutes, lower back, and shoulders.

The Standard for Tight Arch Position:
1. Get set on the floor face down lying flat on your stomach.
2. Pull your feet together and extend your arms straight overhead. Keep your head in a neutral position.
3. Lift your upper and lower half off the floor and squeeze your glutes as you straighten your legs.
4. Point your toes and squeeze your heels together.
5. Hug your ears with straight arms and palms facing towards one another.
6. Make sure your spine stays in a neutral position.

When your feet and heels are not pulled together, your posterior chain and glutes are not as tight as they could be. Tighter equals lighter, which helps prepare you for skills like handstands, pull-ups, and so much more. Like the hollow body position, the tight arch position is about maintaining control and tension throughout your entire body.

Want tips and instructions on bodyweight movements? I've created an appendix to this book that includes a whole bunch of bodyweight movement descriptions, progressions, and modifications, plus access to video demonstrations and photos. Visit the Resources at the end of this book for a link to download the appendix.

THOUGHTS AND MINDSET TIPS

Your mindset shapes how you approach challenges, handle stress, and ultimately, how you live your life. Developing a strong mindset doesn't happen overnight. It's a process, a practice, and, most importantly, a choice you make every single day.

Over the years, I've discovered three simple yet powerful tools that have helped me, as well as my clients, shift toward a healthier, more resilient mindset. Here they are!

Daily Quiet Time

One of the most underrated tools for shifting your mindset is creating quiet time for yourself every day. Quiet time doesn't mean you have to sit in complete silence (unless you want to). It's more about carving out space to pause, reflect, and reset. Quiet time helps calm your mind, reduce stress, and create clarity—especially on busy, overwhelming days.

Some ways to incorporate quiet time:

- Take a 15-minute walk outside. The combination of movement, fresh air, and sunlight is incredibly grounding, plus it's a great way to stack SHIFTS together for more impact.
- Sit with your eyes closed and focus on deep breathing for five to ten minutes.
- Listen to calming music, a guided meditation, or an audiobook that inspires you.
- Engage in a creative activity like journaling, painting, or even doodling.

- Do something soothing, like soaking in a warm bath or spending time in a sauna.

The goal is to step away from the noise of life and give yourself a moment to breathe and reconnect. These small, intentional breaks create a foundation for a calmer, more focused mindset.

Affirmations

The way you talk to yourself matters. Affirmations are a powerful way to rewrite the negative scripts that often play in our minds and replace them with positive, empowering thoughts. Over time and with consistency, the positive, empowering thoughts start to sink in, and you begin to internalize those truths.

If you're not familiar with using affirmations, start small. Pick one or two affirmations that resonate with you, such as:

"I am strong. I am capable. I am resilient."

"I can handle anything that comes my way. Everything I need is already within me."

"Every day, I'm becoming the best version of myself."

Once you've chosen your affirmations, say them out loud. Whether it's in the mirror, in the car, or during your workout, speaking affirmations out loud helps reinforce them in your mind. Personally, I'm an in-the-car affirmations girl, and it's become part of my daily routine to practice my affirmations on my way to client sessions.

Repeat your affirmations daily. The more often you say them, the more they'll shape your thoughts and beliefs. Just as fitness strengthens your mindset and not just your muscles, affirmations are another great tool to build and develop your mindset muscle. The more you practice affirmations, the stronger your mindset will become.

Gratitude Journaling

Gratitude has an incredible ability to shift your mindset, especially on days when life feels heavy or overwhelming. When you focus on what you're grateful for, you retrain your brain to see the good while shifting your nervous system toward a state of balance and optimal functioning instead of dwelling on difficult challenges.

Practicing gratitude positively alters your brain's neurochemistry, increasing dopamine and serotonin levels. It also engages neural pathways linked to high frequency brain states associated with well-being, emotional regulation, high emotional and physiological resilience, empathy, joy, clarity, and calm.[1] Studies show that people who practice gratitude are more likely to engage in healthy behaviors like exercise and regular checkups.[2]

So how do you incorporate more gratitude into your day? I recommend keeping a gratitude journal and adding journaling to your morning or nighttime routine. Getting started with gratitude journaling is simple. Grab a journal or notebook and a pen. I recommend getting a journal specifically to use as your gratitude journal. Over time, you'll build a collection of positive moments to look back on whenever you need a mental boost.

At the beginning or end of each day, write down three things you're grateful for. These don't have to be big, life-changing things. Practicing gratitude for the little things can be as impactful as celebrating the big milestones.

If you're grateful for the sunshine on your walk today, a text from a friend who made you smile, or making it through a challenging workout, jot those items down. Those are wonderful things to express gratitude for.

Then take a moment to reflect on why each of those things matters to you. Taking a moment to connect emotionally to your gratitude makes it even more impactful.

SUNSHINE TIPS: SOAK IT UP!

The beauty of sunshine is that it's free and readily available (unless you live somewhere with limited daylight, like Alaska in winter). Here are some simple ways to incorporate sunshine into your life and make it a part of your daily routine:

Start Your Day Outside. If possible, spend five to ten minutes outside in the morning to help set your circadian rhythm. Even stepping outside with your morning coffee or doing some yoga flow in the early morning sunlight can make a difference, and it can double as quiet time, too!

Skip the Sunscreen for a Few Minutes. To fully absorb the benefits of vitamin D, expose your skin to direct sunlight without sunscreen for 10–20 minutes a day. After that, it's important to protect your skin by applying safe, non-toxic sun protection without harsh chemicals or by wearing protective clothing. But those few minutes of unfiltered sunlight are crucial for maximum benefits.

Get Creative. Whether it's a walk during your lunch break, yoga on your porch, or reading a book in the park, find ways to enjoy the sun that align with your lifestyle. Remember, even on overcast days, being outside is still a great idea, and you don't have to get full sun to reap its benefits.

Make It a Family Activity. Involve your loved ones! Go for a bike ride, have a picnic, or play outside with your kids. These activities not only get you moving, but also allow you to soak in some sunshine while creating lasting memories.

FINAL THOUGHTS ON SHIFTS TIPS

These tips are some of my favorite ways to get started implementing SHIFTS pillars into your life, but they're by no means the only ways. Remember, the most important thing is to choose one pillar to focus on and start.

Choose something you can be consistent with, track your progress, and make adjustments as you go. When you feel you've created a new healthy habit, add another habit and repeat. There's no limit to the amount of progress you can make when you start where you are, show up for yourself consistently, and take action!

[1]Glen R. Fox., Jonas Kaplan, Hanna Damasio, and Antonio Damasio, "Neural Correlates of Gratitude," *Frontiers in Psychology* 6 (September 30, 2015): 1491. https://doi.org/10.3389/fpsyg.2015.01491.

[2] Robert A. Emmons and Michael E. McCullough, "Counting Blessings Versus Burdens: An Experimental Investigation of Gratitude and Subjective Well-Being in Daily Life," *Journal of Personality and Social Psychology* 84, no. 2 (2003): 377–389. https://doi.org/10.1037/0022-3514.84.2.377.

CONCLUSION

L ifelong fitness and wellness is achieved through small, sustainable action taken consistently over time. This book shows you how to build the lifestyle you want where you can live strong, healthy, and happy long term. With the SHIFTS Framework, you can shape your journey in a way that works for you, one habit at a time. The only thing left is to DO it.

This book isn't about quick fixes or unsustainable extremes. Instead, as we worked our way through the pages together, we focused on what truly works: consistent action, a strong mindset, and the SHIFTS Framework.

Movement is Medicine

Fitness is for everyone, and no matter where you're starting from, you can build a stronger, healthier, and happier version of yourself by simply showing up and moving daily. Movement is about more than achieving a number on the scale. It's about freedom, longevity, and quality of life.

The Key to Lifelong Wellness

We broke down the six fundamental SHIFTS—Sleep, Hydration, Intake, Fitness, Thoughts, and Sunshine—and we explored how these simple, science-backed pillars work together to fuel your success. As you bring all of these ideas together for the first time, let's take a quick look back at how everything builds as we move through the SHIFTS Framework.

Sleep: Prioritizing sleep supports muscle recovery, mental clarity, and overall resilience.

Hydration: Drinking enough water is essential to energy, recovery, and daily function.

Intake: Sustainable nutrition means fueling your body with whole foods, prioritizing protein, and reducing unnecessary sugar without deprivation or guilt.

Fitness: Strength isn't just about lifting weights; it's about training for life. Whether you're running with your kids, lifting groceries, or training for competition—movement matters.

Thoughts: Your mindset is your strongest muscle. Training your brain to embrace challenges, push through discomfort, and feed your inner cheerleader is as important as training your body.

Sunshine: Natural light, fresh air, and time outdoors are simple but powerful tools for mood, immunity, and overall well-being.

Consistency is the Ultimate Game-Changer

Progress doesn't come from perfection. It comes from consistency. Choose to show up every day, even when it's hard, even when life is busy, and even when you don't feel like it. Small, intentional efforts add up over time and lead to massive, lifelong transformation.

You Are Capable of More Than You Know

If there's one thing I want you to take away from this book, it's this: You are stronger than you think. You are capable of more than you give yourself credit for. And you are absolutely worthy of the time, effort, and energy it takes to invest in your health and well-being.

Living strong, healthy, and happy is not just for athletes or fitness professionals—it's for parents, business owners, students, and retirees. It's for people with busy lives, demanding schedules, and responsibilities. It's for YOU.

You don't need permission to take control of your health and fitness. You don't need to wait for the "perfect time." You just need to decide that you are worth the effort and take the first step.

Your journey doesn't end here. In fact, this is where the real work begins! As you move forward, I encourage you to:

Start small: Pick one SHIFTS principle to focus on this week and implement it consistently.

Track your progress: Use the tools in this book, journaling, or a fitness tracker to see how your daily actions add up.

Keep learning and growing: Fitness and wellness are lifelong pursuits. Stay curious, stay open, and continue evolving.

Give yourself grace: Progress isn't linear. There will be setbacks, challenges, and moments when you want to quit. Keep showing up. You owe it to your future self to continue forward.

Find support: Surround yourself with people who uplift you, whether that's a coach, a training partner, or a positive community.

Real People, Real Results

I want to leave you with one last story about my client, Monique. She was looking for a way to get stronger and build lean muscle so she could maintain her weight and stay healthy and fit for life. Here's what happened as we started working together and implementing the SHIFTS Framework:

> When I turned 40, I felt like it became much more difficult to lose or maintain my weight. I went to a nutritionist, and she recommended that I see a personal trainer—not just to focus on losing weight, but to build strength and muscle. That's when I started working with Nicole.
>
> At first, it was really difficult and challenging. The workouts pushed me in ways I wasn't used to, but Nicole kept me accountable and made sure I was training safely. I always feel confident that I won't get hurt, and with her guidance, I push myself to lift weights and try movements I never would have attempted on my own. Over time, I've not only become stronger physically, but also mentally. I feel more empowered, and I now know that if I've done it once, I can do it again.
>
> In my experience, the biggest game changer has been fitness. Just looking at everything Nicole does as a mom and a woman over 40 is incredibly inspiring. Seeing her

strength and dedication motivates me to push myself in ways I never thought possible. I also like to follow her nutritional cues, but I feel I still need more guidance and motivation in that area. It's something I continue to work on, along with improving my water intake and sleep habits. One thing I truly appreciate is the special emphasis on sunshine and outdoor activities, always incorporating movement with friends and family. That has been a great reminder for me to stay active in ways that feel enjoyable and sustainable.

Life now feels completely different from when I first started this journey. I feel stronger, more energized, and more confident in my body and what it can do. One of the biggest transformations has been in how I see myself. I've learned to embrace my body with kindness and appreciate my strength. I also understand that this is a process—it takes time, effort, and consistency, and it never really gets "easy," but that's what makes it so rewarding.

I love that I'm able to lift heavy weights and that my kids see they have a strong, healthy mother. It makes me proud to be an example of consistency for my husband and family, and I love knowing that I can inspire my friends to take care of themselves, too.

One of the goals I'm most proud of is the 5K I run with Nicole every year. I've never been a fan of running, and my past experiences with 5Ks weren't exactly fun. But since she invited me to be part of this tradition with her community, I've felt empowered and supported, and each year, I feel stronger and faster.

There's still work to do, but looking back, I'm so proud of how far I've come—and I'm excited to see what's next!

READY TO TAKE THE NEXT STEP?

How about you? Like Monique, do you want training, accountability, and support from me as you implement the SHIFTS Framework in your life? I have coaching programs both in person and online so you can work with me from anywhere in the world.

I individually design programs specific to each client and their unique needs and goals. They choose how many days per week they want programming, and they access it through a private platform online where they can track their progress, get feedback, and ask questions. You also receive one-on-one custom nutrition coaching, full access to the True Coach logging and tracking system, remote coaching video analysis, one-on-one monthly consultations, and my entire video library with movement demonstrations and coaching tutorials.

Visit https://NicoleZapoli.com/remote-coaching/ to apply. I am so pumped and ready to help you build your strongest, healthiest, happiest life!

You Are the Architect of Your Life

At the end of the day, no one can do this but YOU.

But you don't have to do it alone.

I believe in you. I believe in your strength, your resilience, and your ability to create a life that reflects the strongest, healthiest, and happiest version of YOU.

The only way is through. At this point, you have everything you need to move forward with confidence.

Now, let's go live our strongest, live our healthiest, live our happiest lives possible!

I'll be right alongside you cheering for you every step of the way!

–Coach Z

RESOURCES

I want to make getting started as simple and easy as possible. That's why I've created a special bonus section on my website for book readers only that contains downloadable resources, video demonstrations, recipes, trackers, and more! **Visit https://nicolezapoli.com/book-resources/ to access all the resources below, and enter your information for access.** You'll receive a welcome email with the link where you can access all the bonus content.

Chapter 4: Showing Up for Yourself

Create Your Avatar Worksheet
Describe the ultimate version of you then determine the action steps you'll take to get there with this downloadable PDF guide.

Chapter 6: Shifting Gears

Spren App for Body Composition
Want a quick and easy way to monitor your body composition? Download the Spren app and turn your phone into a validated health lab for your physiology where you can track your body fat, resting metabolic heart rate, lean mass, and overall body composition health score.

Section 7.3: Intake and Nutrition

Phase 1 Nutrition Guide
Need an overview of foundational nutrition basics? The Phase 1 Nutrition Guide breaks down how to optimize your water, food, function and energy so you can fuel your body and achieve your fitness and wellness goals.

Phase 1 Nutrition "In a Nutshell"
A shorter grab-and-go version of the Phase 1 Nutrition Guide. Print it off and hang it on your fridge for fast reference.

Chapter 9: Starting Off Right

7-Day NZ Fitness Program
Jumpstart your training with seven days of free programming, including training videos, recovery, and more!

Chapter 10: Tracking Your SHIFTS

NZ Fitness and Wellness Questionnaire
Assessing where you are right now will help you determine your best starting point. My NZ Fitness and Wellness Questionnaire, a downloadable PDF, is a great place to start. This is the same questionnaire my clients fill out when we begin working together.

SHIFTS Tracker
Ready to track your SHIFTS? This downloadable, printable tracker makes it easy to track your sleep, hydration, intake, fitness, thoughts, and sunshine every day so you can create new healthy habits!

Chapter 11: Best Tips for Core Shifts

NZ Meals Curated Menu
Want help with healthy meals? My NZ Meals partnership with Territory makes it easy to have locally sourced and created fresh—never frozen—meals curated by me from local chefs delivered straight to your door. Available in 27 states, these meals are free of common allergens to reduce inflammation, allergic reactions, and food sensitivities. No gluten, no dairy, no grains. Visit https://meals.nicolezapoli.com/menu?discountCode=MEALPREPWITHNZ to get $25 off your first order.

NZ Nutrition App
Tired of not knowing what to eat, when to eat it, and how much? Take the guesswork out of your nutrition and get the results you have been looking for with a free 14-day trial of my customized NZ Nutrition App. https://NicoleZapoli.com/nz-fit-app/

60 Minute Strength + Stretch Session
You can find this free session on the Resources page of my website.

Bodyweight Movement Appendix and Glossary of Fitness Terms

If you're ready to take things to the next level, I've also created a bonus section as an appendix to this book that details bodyweight movements based on functional gymnastics, complete with photos and videos. You'll also find a step by step guide for making your own inexpensive, lightweight, compact, and versatile piece of equipment that is perfect for at home use or travel. This tool pairs with many of the position drills and movement progressions in the movement appendix, giving you even more ways to train effectively with just your bodyweight. It can also be accessed by visiting https://NicoleZapoli.com/book-resources/.

ABOUT NICOLE ZAPOLI

Nicole is a professional fitness and wellness coach, certified personal trainer, athlete, and more! Nicole's passion, purpose, and mission in life is to help empower others to live their strongest, healthiest, happiest lives possible.

Nicole is also a proud mom to two amazing kids, Rylee and Declan, and soulmate to the love of her life, Jon. She loves spending quality time with her family and friends, training, adventuring, traveling, being artsy, painting, listening to music, playing in the ocean, dancing, yoga, and anything outdoors.

Early Life

From as early as 8 years old, Nicole knew she wanted to own her own gym business, be a coach, entrepreneur, and—most importantly—that she wanted to help people when she grew up. As a young girl, she loved how empowering, fun, and awesome it was to feel and BE strong, healthy, and happy. Nicole knew from then on she would be spreading her love and passion for fitness to others for the rest of her life!

Originally from Texas, Nicole began her lifelong fitness journey with dance at the age of 2, gymnastics at 4, and was competing in artistic gymnastics by 6 years old. She later switched to rhythmic gymnastics.

By the age of 14, Nicole had received the opportunity to train at the United States Olympic Training Center and was a four-time Texas State Champion in rhythmic gymnastics, four-time Junior Olympian, and a member of the US Junior Olympic Academic Team.

Following rhythmic gymnastics, she cheered competitively for three years, becoming a three-time All-American cheerleader. Nicole went on to dance and cheer professionally for the NFL Houston Texans and the NBA Houston Rockets along with various other professional dance companies.

Career

Nicole started her first business when she was 19 years old, a mobile gym business, offering in-home personal training as well as cheer, dance, and gymnastics coaching programs at private schools, daycares, and after-school community programs.

A few years later, in 2009, she discovered CrossFit and decided to become a CrossFit Trainer as well as a CrossFit Gymnastics (CFG) Trainer. Soon after that, Nicole was invited to intern and eventually joined the CFG Seminar Team. For the past 14 years, Nicole has had the opportunity to travel the world and teach gymnastics in the functional fitness and CrossFit world both as part of CFG as well as within her own business and brand, NZ Fitness. She has now booked, organized, planned, prepped, taught, coached, and led more than 130 NZ Fitness gymnastics workshops worldwide, as well as over 40 CFG Seminars worldwide.

Nicole has had the opportunity to be part of many fitness community events locally and worldwide while representing several fitness companies as an athlete, ambassador, business owner, seminar coach, etc.

The amount of willingness and dedication to her own personal growth and pushing past her comfort zone is beyond all comprehension. Nicole is proud of herself for having the courage to say yes to new life opportunities.

The honor to receive and say yes to new, amazing life adventures to level up always far outweighs fear!

Nicole eventually opened her own CrossFit affiliate when she was 29 years old and was brought on as a co-owner of another already established CrossFit affiliate when she was 34 years old.

In 2016, Nicole's seventh entrepreneurial venture and business baby, NZ Fitness LLC was born; offering remote online coaching plus custom programming, personal training, virtual personal training, gymnastics workshops, a mobile custom nutrition app, and nutrition coaching support. You can also find NZ Fitness in-person training located throughout the county of San Diego, in homes and outdoors, resort and boutique gyms, CrossFit affiliates, and more!

Nicole's lifelong fitness journey has allowed and continues to allow her endless opportunities to create, grow, learn, build, and evolve as a person, mom, athlete, business owner, and entrepreneur. She is forever grateful for the many people, experiences, adventures, and beyond that have shaped her into who she is today.

·ss Strength and Conditioning

.less training method is designed to build strength, , work capacity, and increase lean body mass so that ·itness clients have the ability to live their strongest, ,thiest, happiest lives possible. All program designs are rived from over 30 years of experience in training and oaching including artistic and rhythmic gymnastics, CFG, bodybuilding, power lifting, tactical training, Olympic weightlifting, yoga and ayurveda, adaptive training, and US Olympic strength and conditioning training and coaching methodologies.

Nicole's top priority is creating a training protocol that revolves around safety via optimal body mechanics, technique, and building a solid movement foundation. She wants her clients progressing across all domains as they continue building their base strength and overall conditioning.

Training Accomplishments

Nicole has also studied, trained, and competed in various sports such as Fitness America, CrossFit, USAW (weightlifting), USPA (powerlifting), PNBA (professional natural bodybuilding). She won Fitness America Texas in 2006 and Fitness America California in 2011 along with receiving the opportunity to be a contestant on American Ninja Warrior in 2013. She is the 2015 USPA California State Champion (48kg) and bench press record holder. She placed in the top 10% fittest ladies in North America in the 2021 CrossFit Games Open and the top 10% fittest ladies in the world in her age group advancing her into the Quarterfinals and the worldwide age group online qualifiers.

Nicole placed in the top 5% fittest ladies in the world in her age group and the top 8% fittest ladies in the 2024 CrossFit Games Individual Open, advancing her into the Quarterfinals and the worldwide age group online qualifiers.

Most recently, Nicole placed in the top 6% fittest ladies in the world in her age group and the top 7% fittest ladies in the 2025 CrossFit Games Individual Open.

Nicole placed first in Sports Model and received Best Presentation at the 2023 INBA Southern California & Armed Forces Championships.

She then went on to place first in Figure at the 2023 PNBA/INBA Zeus Classic where she also received her pro athlete qualification.

She made her pro debut in Figure, received her pro card in Sports Model at the 2023 PNBA/INBA Team USA Championships. Nicole then qualified plus went pro in two categories, Figure and Sports Model, at the 2023 Natural Olympia.

She placed first in Pro Sports Model and second place in Pro Figure at the Mr. & Ms. USA Championships in 2024.

After 42.5 weeks of living that fun, fit pregnancy journey, Nicole gave birth to her second beautiful and healthy baby in December 2022.

In the summer of 2024 she competed in the regional calisthenics competition and placed top three in all events for max strict pull-ups, deficit push-ups, strict dips, sit-ups, and air squats. Resulting in a second overall finish.

Coaching Credentials

Nicole has over 25 years coaching experience and holds multiple coach, trainer, and specialty certifications including:

Conjugate Tactical Course Instructor SME—Bodyweight Movement Specialist

VR Personal Trainer

NASM, Certified Personal Trainer

250 HR RYT Yoga

OPEX CCP L1 Total Coach

OPEX Certified Nutrition Coach

OPEX Certified Life Coach

OPEX Certified in Assessment & Program Design

OPEX Certified in Business Systems

CrossFit Level 2 Trainer

CrossFit Level 1 Trainer

CrossFit Gymnastics Trainer

CrossFit Kids Trainer

CrossFit Football Trainer

CrossFit Certified Judge

Physical Fitness Specialist, Cooper Institute

Certified Nurse Assistant

CPR, AED Certified

www.ingramcontent.com/pod-product-compliance
Lightning Source LLC
Chambersburg PA
CBHW062126020426

42335CB00013B/1116